American Medical Association

Physicians dedicated to the health of America

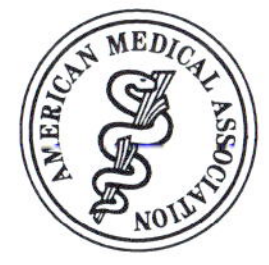

Trends in US Health Care

Fourth edition

Additional copies may be ordered from:
Order Dept. OP190295
American Medical Association
For order information call toll-free 800 621-8335
ISBN 0-89970-735-1

BP71:95-0110:2M:9/95

Introduction

This, the fourth edition of *Trends in US Health Care,* continues the tradition of providing a ready source of comprehensive data on health in the United States. In an era when health policy and health system issues are receiving heightened attention, the publication of an updated volume is particularly timely. Experienced users will find that the best features of previous editions have been retained, while many new exhibits have been added. The objective of *Trends* remains as it always has: To present readers with a variety of statistics and presentation formats amenable for easy adaption to particular needs.

I wish to acknowledge the contributions of two individuals. James W. Moser, PhD supervised the editorial aspects of the project. Sarah L. Gordon was principally responsible for research, data collection, and tabulations.

James F. Rodgers, PhD
Director
AMA Center for Health Policy Research
August 1995

Table of contents

The nation's health

Statistics on the population at large: birth rates, death rates and population growth.
International comparisons are included for most variables.

Numbers that indicate the prevalence and recent trends of certain illnesses and health threatening situations in the population.

Health care delivery

Information on the delivery of health services by physicians and other health care professionals—
with data on productivity, income, liability, and education.

Changes in the hospital system as indicated by traditional utilization measures. International comparisons are included.

List of exhibits

Vital statistics

Population

Life expectancy at birth

Birth rates

Infant mortality rates

Medical practice and health workforce

Hospitals

The nation's health

Vital statistics

Population

Exhibit 1. **Resident population (in thousands) and percentage distribution by age and race**

	1950	1960	1970	1980	1990	1993	1994	1995	2000	2020	2040
Total population	150,697	179,323	203,236	226,546	248,710	257,908	260,662	263,434	276,241	300,431	325,942
Age structure											
· Under 15	26.9%	31.1%	28.5%	22.6%	21.7%	22.0%	–	22.1%	21.7%	20.1%	19.9%
· 15-35	30.4%	26.1%	29.7%	35.1%	32.2%	30.7%	–	29.6%	27.5%	27.1%	26.7%
· 35-65	34.6%	33.5%	32.0%	31.0%	33.6%	34.6%	–	35.5%	38.0%	39.4%	37.1%
· over 65	8.1%	9.2%	9.8%	11.3%	12.5%	12.6%	–	12.8%	12.8%	13.3%	16.4%
Racial distribution											
· White	89.3%	88.6%	87.6%	85.9%	83.9%	83.3%	–	82.9%	81.9%	80.0%	78.2%
· Black	9.9%	10.5%	11.1%	11.8%	12.3%	12.5%	–	12.6%	12.8%	13.4%	13.9%
· Other race	0.7%	0.9%	1.3%	2.3%	3.9%	4.3%	–	4.5%	5.3%	6.6%	7.9%
· Hispanic*	–	–	–	6.4%	9.0%	9.7%	–	10.2%	11.3%	13.5%	15.7%

Figures for 1950-1990 are as of April 1 of that year. For 1991 and beyond, figures are as of July 1 of that year.

Age and racial distribution figures are provisional for 1993 and later years.

* Persons of Hispanic origin may be of any race.

Source: Bureau of the Census

Exhibit 2. **International population comparisons (in thousands)**

Ten largest countries in 1994			Other 1994 populations	
1	Mainland China	1,190,431	Austria	7,955
2	India	919,903	Belgium	10,063
3	United States	260,714	Canada	28,114
4	Indonesia	200,410	Denmark	5,188
5	Brazil	158,739	France	57,840
6	Russia	149,609	Germany	81,088
7	Pakistan	128,856	Ireland	3,539
8	Bangladesh	125,149	Italy	58,138
9	Japan	125,107	Luxembourg	402
10	Nigeria	98,091	Mexico	92,202
			Netherlands	15,368
			Norway	4,315
			Spain	39,303
			Sweden	8,778
			Switzerland	7,040
			United Kingdom	58,135

Source: Bureau of the Census

Life expectancy at birth

Exhibit 3. Life expectancy at birth (in years)

	1950*	1960*	1970	1980	1985	1990	1991	1992+	1993+
All races									
· Total	68.2	69.7	70.8	73.7	74.7	75.4	75.5	75.7	75.5
· Male	65.6	66.6	67.1	70.0	71.1	71.8	72.0	72.3	72.1
· Female	71.1	73.1	74.8	77.4	78.2	78.8	78.9	79.0	78.9
White									
· Total	69.1	70.6	71.7	74.4	75.3	76.1	76.3	76.5	76.3
· Male	66.5	67.4	68.0	70.7	71.8	72.7	72.9	73.2	73.0
· Female	72.2	74.1	75.6	78.1	78.7	79.4	79.6	79.7	79.5
Black									
· Total	60.7	63.2	64.1	68.1	69.3	69.1	69.3	69.8	69.3
· Male	58.9	60.7	60.0	63.8	65.0	64.5	64.6	65.5	64.7
· Female	62.7	65.9	68.3	72.5	73.4	73.6	73.8	73.9	73.7

Life expectancy at age 65

	1950*	1960*	1970	1980	1985	1990	1991	1992+	1993+
All races	13.9	14.3	15.2	16.4	16.7	17.2	17.4	17.5	17.3

* Includes births and deaths of nonresidents of the United States.

+ Provisional.

Source: National Center for Health Statistics

Exhibit 4. **International life expectancy comparisons, 1990**

Country	Years		Change since 1985	
	Women	*Men*	*Women*	*Men*
Austria	79.2	72.6	1.8	2.2
Belgium	78.2	72.0	0.4	0.2
Canada	80.8	74.0	0.8	0.9
France	81.8	73.4	1.7	1.6
Germany	79.2	69.3	0.9	−0.2
Greece	79.8	74.6	1.3	1.1
Italy	80.4	73.6	1.6	1.4
Japan	82.5	76.2	1.5	1.2
Netherlands	80.3	73.9	0.4	0.8
Sweden	80.8	74.8	1.0	1.0
Switzerland	81.0	74.0	0.6	0.5
United Kingdom	78.9	73.2	1.3	1.3
United States	78.8	71.8	0.6	0.7

Source: World Health Organization

Birth rates

Exhibit 5. **Birth rates: All races, white and black** (Live births per 1,000 population)

	1950	1960	1970	1980	1990	1991	1992+	1993+
Total	24.1	23.7	18.4	15.9	16.7	16.3	16.0	15.7
White	23.0	22.7	17.4	14.9	15.5	15.4	15.0	na
Black	na	31.9	25.3	22.1	23.8	21.9	21.3	na

+Provisional.
na—not available
Source: National Center for Health Statistics

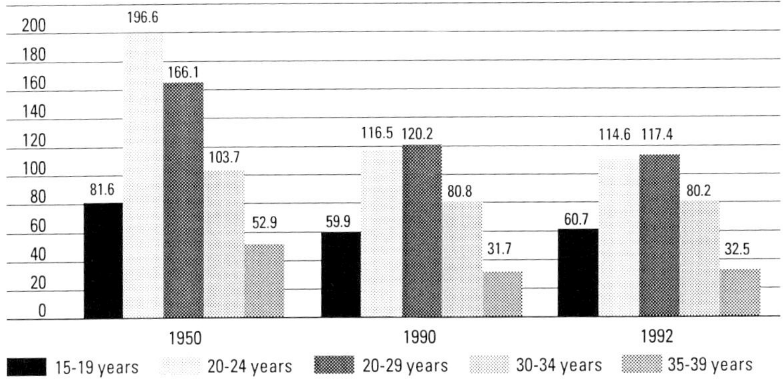

Source: National Center for Health Statistics

Birth rates, continued

Exhibit 7. International birth rate comparisons, 1992
(Live births per 1,000 population)

High growth		Low growth	
Niger	55.0	Greece	10.5
Mali	51.8	Japan	10.5
Yemen	50.7	Italy	10.8
Malawi	50.4	Germany	11.0
Rwanda	49.2	Spain	11.1
Uganda	48.8	Austria	11.4
Burkina	48.4	Belgium	11.7
Zaire	48.4	Switzerland	12.2
Benin	47.7	Denmark	12.5
Cote d'Ivoire	46.5	Netherlands	12.6
Somalia	46.0	Russia	12.7
Tanzania	45.5	France	13.1
Angola	45.4	United Kingdom	13.4
Afghanistan	43.5	Sweden	13.5
Nigeria	43.5	Canada	14.1
Pakistan	42.2	United States	16.0
		Mainland China	18.1

Source: Bureau of the Census

Exhibit 8. **Infant mortality: All races, white and black (per thousand)**

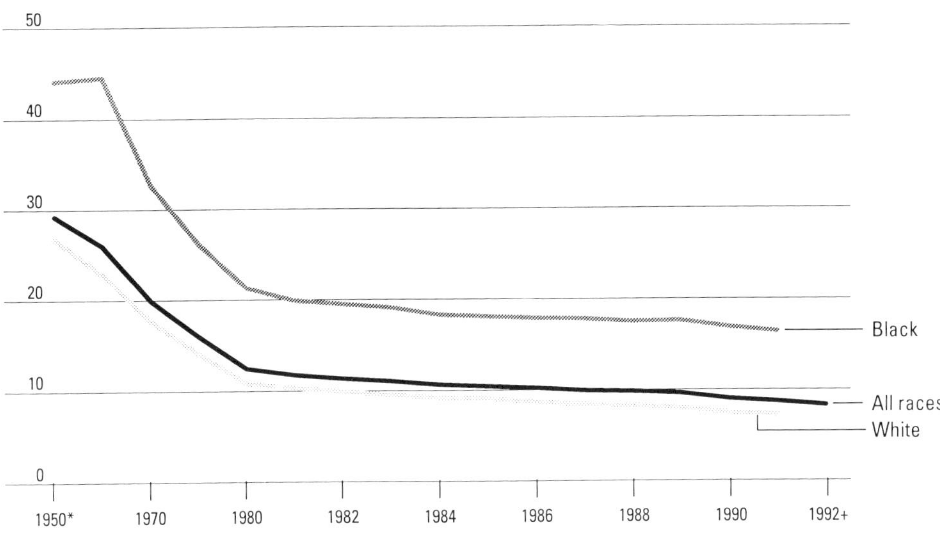

Infant mortality rates, continued

All races	1950*	1960*	1970	1980	1990	1991	1992+	1993+
Infant	29.2	26.0	20.0	12.6	9.2	8.9	8.5	8.3
Neonatal	20.5	18.7	15.1	8.5	5.8	5.6	5.4	5.4

Infant mortality rate refers to deaths of infants before the first birthday.
Neonatal mortality refers to deaths of infants under 28 days old.
+Provisional.
* Includes births and deathos of nonresidents of the United States.
Source: National Center for Health Statistics

Exhibit 9. International infant mortality comparisons, 1990

Country	Infant mortality (per thousand)	Country	Infant mortality (per thousand)
Japan	4.6	Austria	7.8
Sweden	6.0	United Kingdom	7.9
Switzerland	6.8	Belgium	7.9
Canada	6.8	Italy	8.5
Netherlands	7.1	United States	9.2
Germany	7.3	US White	7.7
France	7.3	US Black	17.0

Source: World Health Organization

Exhibit 10. **Age-adjusted death rates, by race and sex (deaths per 100,000 resident population)**

	1950*	1960*	1970	1980	1990	1991	1992+	1993+
All Races	840.5	760.9	714.3	585.8	520.2	513.7	504.9	514.0
White								
· Men	963.1	917.7	893.4	745.3	644.3	634.4	620.9	631.2
· Women	645.0	555.0	501.7	411.1	369.9	366.3	360.2	366.1
Black								
· Men	1373.1	1246.1	1318.6	1112.8	1061.3	1048.8	1026.1	1051.1
· Women	1106.7	916.9	814.4	631.1	581.6	575.1	570.0	583.1

* Includes deaths of nonresidents of the United States.
+ Provisional data.
Source: National Center for Health Statistics.

Death rates, continued

Exhibit 11. **Ten leading causes of death, 1993**

Rank	Cause	Death rate per 100,000 population	% of total deaths
1	Diseases of the heart	286.9	32.6
2	Malignant neoplasms	205.8	23.4
3	Cerebrovascular disease	58.1	6.6
4	Chronic obstructive pulmonary disease	39.2	4.5
5	Unintentional injuries	34.4	3.9
6	Pneumonia/influenza	31.7	3.6
7	Diabetes mellitus	21.4	2.4
8	Human immunodeficiency virus	14.9	1.7
9	Suicide	12.1	1.4
10	Homicide and legal intervention	9.9	1.1

Source: National Center for Health Statistics

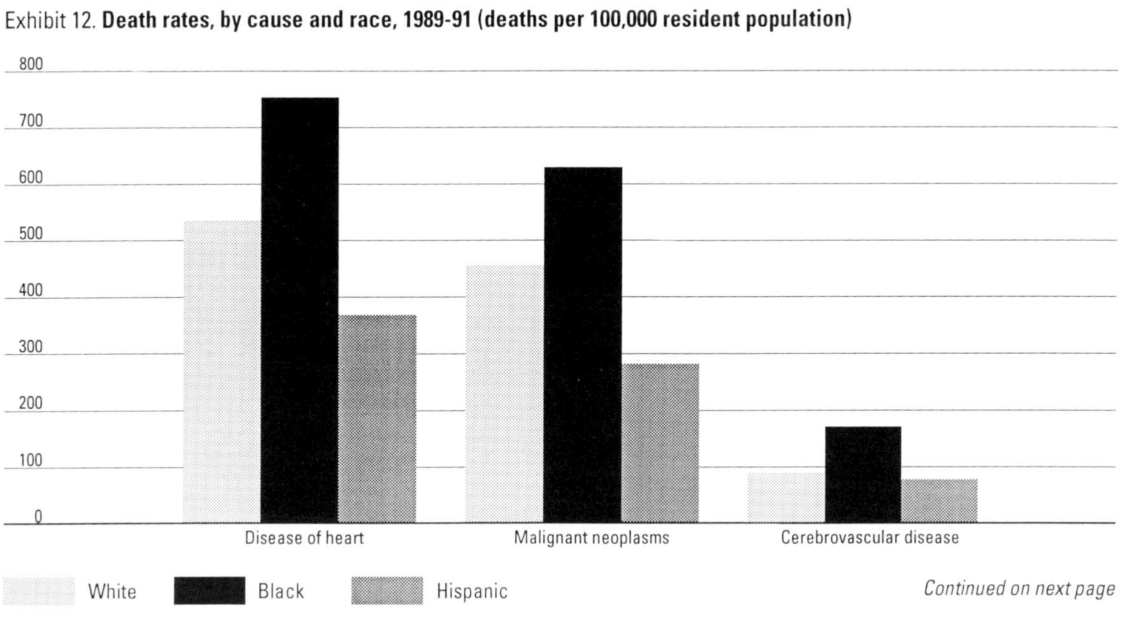

Continued on next page

Exhibit 12. **Death rates, by cause and race, 1989-91, continued (deaths per 100,000 resident population)**

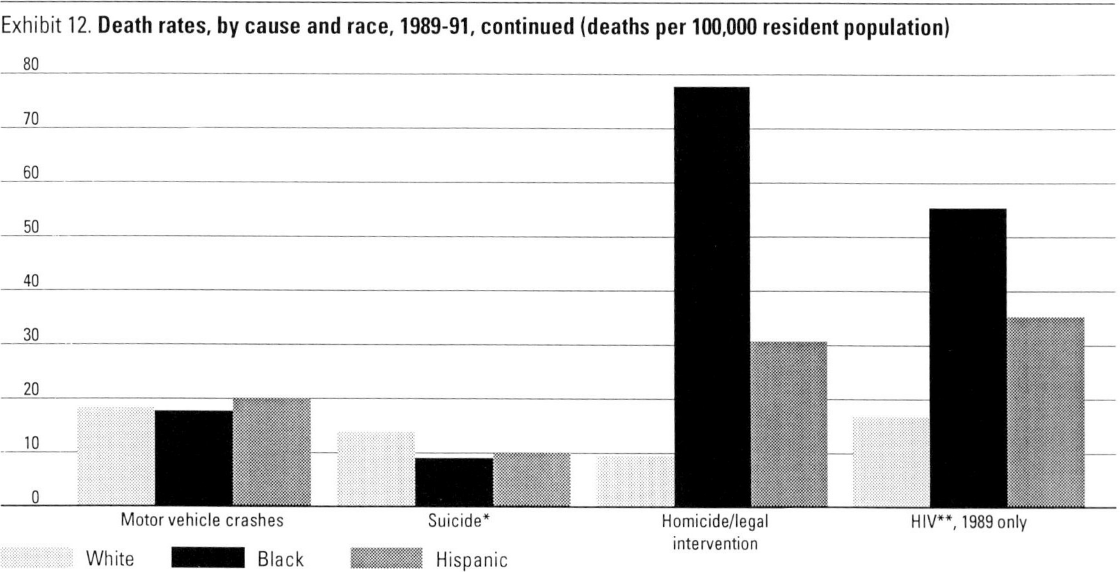

Note: Rates are for age 45 years and over, age adjusted, unless otherwise indicated.
* Figures include age-adjusted death rates for 15-24 year-old individuals only.
** Figure includes age-adjusted death rates for 25-44 year-olds only.
Source: National Center for Health Statistics

The nation's health

Threats to health

Exhibit 13. **Selected notifiable disease rates**

Number of cases per 100,000 population*

Sexually transmitted diseases	*1960*	*1970*	*1980*	*1985*	*1987*	*1989*	*1991*	*1992*
Syphilis	68.78	45.26	30.51	28.50	35.81	44.94	51.69	45.30
Gonorrhea	145.33	297.22	444.99	384.28	323.14	297.36	249.48	201.60
Chancroid	0.94	0.70	0.35	0.87	2.07	1.90	1.40	0.80
Granuloma Inguinale	0.17	0.06	0.02	0.02	0.01	0.00	0.01	0.00
Lymphogranuloma Venereum	0.47	0.30	0.09	0.10	0.13	0.08	0.19	0.10

Other notifiable diseases

	1960	1970	1980	1985	1987	1989	1991	1992
AIDS	–	–	–	4.75	11.30	15.20	17.20	17.80
Diphtheria	0.51	0.21	0.00	0.00	0.00	0.00	0.00	0.00
Hepatitis A+	–	27.87	12.84	10.03	10.39	14.43	9.67	9.06
Hepatitis B+	–	4.08	8.39	11.50	10.65	9.43	7.14	6.32
Mumps	–	55.55	3.86	1.30	5.43	2.34	1.72	1.03
Pertussis (Whooping Cough)	8.23	2.08	0.76	1.50	1.16	1.67	1.08	1.60
Poliomyelitis	1.77	0.02	0.00	0.00	0.00	0.00	0.00	0.00
Rubella (German Measles)	–	27.75	1.72	0.26	0.13	0.16	0.56	0.60
Rubeola (Measles)	245.42	23.23	5.96	1.18	1.50	7.33	3.82	0.88
Salmonellosis, excluding Typhoid Fever	3.85	10.84	14.88	27.37	20.92	19.26	19.10	16.04
Shigellosis	6.94	6.79	8.41	7.14	9.80	10.07	9.34	9.38
Tuberculosis	30.83	18.22	12.25	9.30	9.25	9.46	10.42	10.46
Varicella (Chickenpox)	–	–	96.69	123.33	136.68	121.77	135.82	176.54

* The total resident population was used to calculate all rates except sexually transmitted diseases, for which the resident civilian population was used.

+ Reports from New York City are not available for 1985.

Sources: National Center for Health Statistics

Threats to children

Exhibit 14. **Ten leading causes of death for infants under one year of age, 1992**

Cause	Mortality rate (per 100,000 live births)
All causes	851.9
Congenital anomalies	183.2
Sudden infant death syndrome	120.3
Premature or low birthweight	99.3
Respiratory distress	50.8
Maternal complications	35.9
Complications of placenta, cord or membrane	24.4
Perinatal infections	22.2
Accidents and adverse effects	20.1
Hypoxia and birth asphyxia	15.1
Pneumonia and influenza	14.8
Ill defined causes	265.8

Source: National Center for Health Statistics

Exhibit 15. **Vaccination rates for children 19-35 months old, 1992 (percent of children 19-35 months)**

	Race			Poverty status		Location of residence		
	Total	White	Black	Below poverty	At or above poverty	Central city	Remaining MSA areas	Outside MSA
Diptheria-Tetanus-Pertussis (DPT)	83.0	84.8	74.7	79.7	84.6	82.5	84.4	80.7
Polio*	72.4	74.1	62.7	66.6	74.7	74.1	72.6	69.0
Measles containing or MMR**	82.5	83.6	77.9	80.2	84.3	84.5	83.3	77.2
Haemophilus B (HIB)***	66.6	69.2	54.9	58.1	70.5	65.3	67.9	65.8

Notes: *Three doses or more
**Measles-Mumps-Rubella
***One or more doses
Source: National Center for Health Statistics

Exhibit 16. **Incidence of low birthweight*, by race (percentage of all births)**

	1970	1975	1980	1985	1990	1991	1992
All Infants	7.9	7.4	6.8	6.8	7.0	7.1	7.1
White	6.8	6.3	5.7	5.7	5.7	5.8	5.8
Black	13.9	13.1	12.5	12.6	13.3	13.6	13.3

*Less than 2,500 grams
**Based on 100% of birth in select states and 50% sample in all other states.
Source: National Center for Health Statistics

Threats to children, continued

Exhibit 17. **Births to young and unmarried women, by race, 1991**
(Percent of total births)

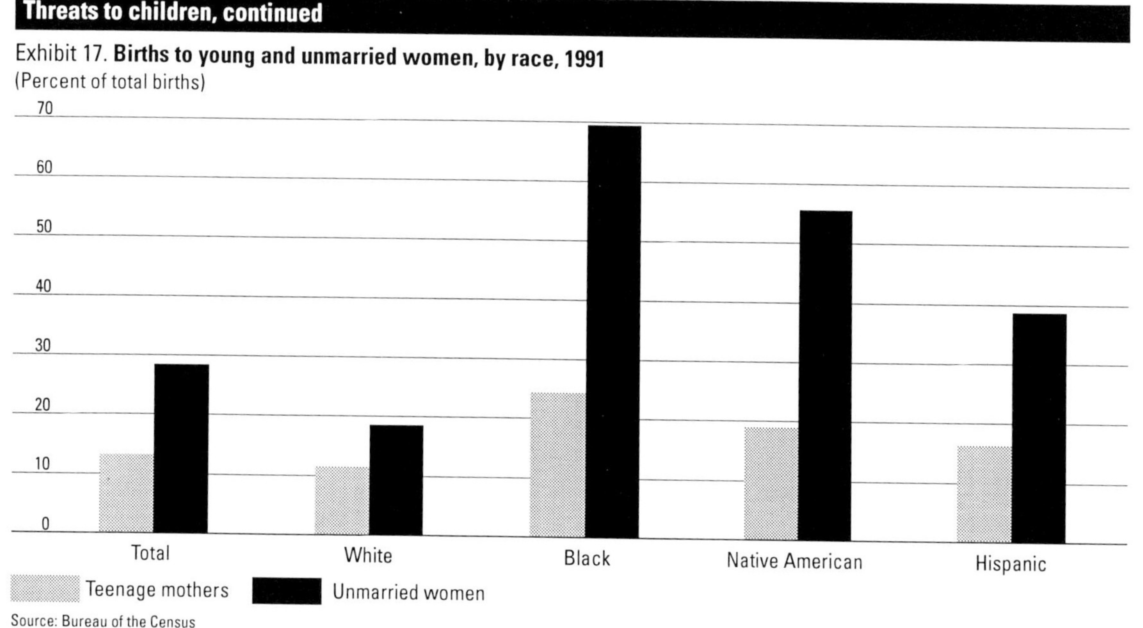

Source: Bureau of the Census

Exhibit 18. **International birth rates to women under 20 years of age, circa 1990 (number of births per 1,000 women)**

Country	Year	All ages	Women 15-19
United States	1989	61.8	59.4
Australia	1990	58.3	22.0
Canada	1989	54.5	24.8
France	1990	54.5	9.1
Germany	1988	43.7	10.3
Italy	1988	39.4	9.6
Japan	1990	38.9	3.6
Netherlands	1990	49.9	8.3
New Zealand	1990	67.2	34.4
Norway	1990	58.0	16.9
Spain	1986	47.1	16.7
Sweden	1989	57.7	12.7
United Kingdom	1990	56.5	33.0

Source: Office of Technology Assessment

HIV/AIDS

Exhibit 19. **AIDS cases reported***

	1985	*1987*	*1988*	*1989*	*1990*	*1991*	*1992*	*1993*	*1994*
Total cases	8,189	21,048	30,648	33,511	41,558	43,574	45,603	103,228	78,126
Children <13 years	129	319	565	592	718	669	744	942	1,017
Adults/adolescents	8,060	20,729	30,083	32,919	40,840	42,905	44,859	102,286	77,109
Distribution of adult/adolescent cases by sex									
Male	94%	92%	90%	90%	89%	87%	87%	84%	82%
Female	6%	8%	10%	10%	11%	13%	13%	16%	18%

*AIDS case reporting definitions were expanded in 1985, 1987 and 1993. This may hinder the comparison of figures over time.
Source: Centers for Disease Control

Exhibit 20. **Deaths from AIDS**

	1985	*1987*	*1988*	*1989*	*1990*	*1991*	*1992*	*1993*
Total Deaths	6,704	15,504	19,263	25,978	27,311	32,573	39,307	41,919
Persons under 13	106	272	293	337	360	349	353	406*
Persons 13 or over	6,598	15,232	18,970	25,641	26,951	32,224	38,954	41,513*

Totals are for the U.S. not including territories.
*Figures indicate deaths of persons under or over the age of 15.
Source: Centers for Disease Control

Exhibit 21. **AIDS cases by state—number of cases and percentage of total cases, 1994**

	Total	Percent		Total	Percent
New York	83,197	19%	Maryland	10,534	2%
California	78,084	18%	Massachusetts	9,254	2%
Florida	43,978	10%	District of Columbia	7,129	2%
Texas	30,712	7%	Louisiana	6,611	1%
New Jersey	25,089	6%	Ohio	6,509	1%
Illinois	14,255	3%	Virginia	6,318	1%
Pennsylvania	12,754	3%	Michigan	6,240	1%
Georgia	12,228	3%	Washington	5,922	1%

Source: Centers for Disease Control

HIV/AIDS (continued)

Exhibit 22. **AIDS cases, case-fatality rates and deaths occuring during interval, by half year**

		Adults/adolescents		Children <13 years			Adults/adolescents		Children <13 years	
		Cases diagnosed	Fatality rates	Cases diagnosed	Fatality rates		Cases diagnosed	Fatality rates	Cases diagnosed	Fatality rates
Before 1981		88	87.5	8	75.0					
1981	Jan-June	102	90.2	10	80.0	July-Dec	199	92.5	6	83.3
1982	Jan-June	420	93.3	14	92.9	July-Dec	723	91.1	16	87.5
1983	Jan-June	1,331	93.8	32	100.0	July-Dec	1,690	93.8	43	90.7
1984	Jan-June	2,649	93.4	52	86.5	July-Dec	3,481	93.6	63	87.3
1985	Jan-June	5,085	92.6	107	80.4	July-Dec	6,506	92.7	136	83.1
1986	Jan-June	8,622	91.8	142	83.8	July-Dec	10,192	92.1	193	76.2
1987	Jan-June	13,435	90.9	226	77.0	July-Dec	14,840	88.9	267	72.3
1988	Jan-June	17,259	86.7	262	68.7	July-Dec	17,759	86.7	246	64.7
1989	Jan-June	20,702	83.1	371	63.1	July-Dec	21,075	81.5	346	65.8

1990	Jan-June	23,706	78.3	379	60.2	July-Dec	23,298	75.4	395	50.6
1991	Jan-June	27,533	70.8	392	50.8	July-Dec	29,599	65.4	381	45.9
1992	Jan-June	35,524	55.7	458	42.1	July-Dec	38,330	47.3	412	42.0
1993	Jan-June	39,077	33.1	394	32.7	July-Dec	31,363	25.4	379	29.6
1994	Jan-June	28,176	15.9	270	20.0	July-Dec	12,555	8.3	109	11.9

Source: Centers for Disease Control

Alcohol, Smoking and Substance Use

Exhibit 23. **Per capita ethanol consumption by adults (in gallons)**

Beverage	1975	1980	1985	1990	1991	1992
Beer	30.6	36.6	34.6	34.9	33.2	32.7
Wine+	2.2	3.2	3.5	2.9	2.7	2.7
Spirits	3.0	3.0	2.6	2.2	2.0	2.0
Total#	35.7	42.8	40.7	40.0	37.8	37.4

+ Beginning in 1983, includes wine coolers.
# Figures may not add due to rounding.
Source: United States Department of Agriculture

Exhibit 24. **Percentages of adults reporting themselves as current cigarette smokers**

	1965	*1974*	*1979*	*1983*	*1985*	*1987*	*1990*	*1992+*
All persons 18 *	42.3	37.2	33.5	32.2	30.0	28.7	25.4	26.4
All males 18 and over*	51.6	42.9	37.2	34.7	32.1	31.0	28.0	28.2
· 18-24 years	54.1	42.1	35.0	32.9	28.0	28.2	26.6	28.0
· 25-34 years	60.7	50.5	43.9	38.8	38.2	34.8	31.6	32.8
· 35-44 years	58.2	51.0	41.8	41.0	37.6	36.6	34.5	32.9
· 45-64 years	51.9	42.6	39.3	35.9	33.4	33.5	29.3	28.6
· 65+ years	28.5	24.8	20.9	22.0	19.6	17.2	14.6	16.1
All females 18 and over*	34.0	32.5	30.3	29.9	28.2	26.7	23.1	24.8
· 18-24 years	38.1	34.1	33.8	35.5	30.4	26.1	22.5	24.9
· 25-34 years	43.7	38.8	33.7	32.6	32.0	31.8	28.2	30.1
· 35-44 years	43.7	39.8	37.0	33.8	31.5	29.6	24.8	27.3
· 45-64 years	32.0	33.4	30.7	31.0	29.9	28.6	24.8	26.1
· 65+ years	9.6	12.0	13.2	13.1	13.5	13.7	11.5	12.4

* Age-adjusted.

+ Not strictly comparable with earlier years. 1992 definition includes occasional smokers, whereas earlier-year definition excluded them.

Source: National Center for Health Statistics

Exhibit 25. **Self reported drug use among high school seniors**

(Percentage of all respondents reporting ever having used marijuana or cocaine in their life)

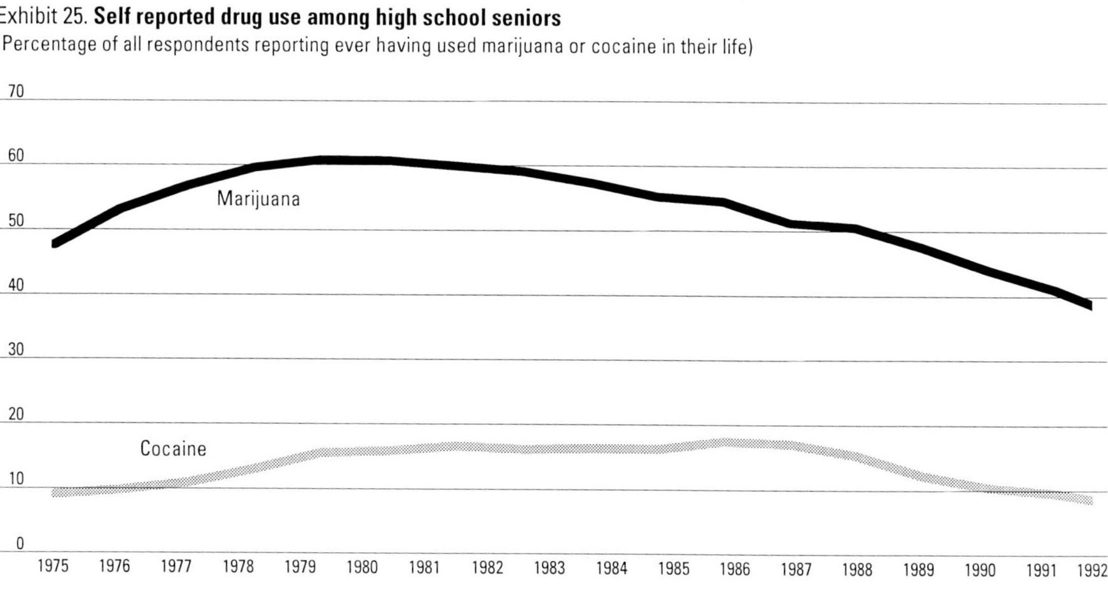

Source: Monitoring the Future Survey

Exhibit 26. **Crime victimization by type of crime, 1992**

	Number of incidents	% of total
All types	33,649,340	100%
Personal crime	18,831,980	56
Violence	**6,621,140**	**20**
· Rape	140,930	0
· Robbery	1,225,510	4
· Assault	5,254,690	16
Theft	**12,210,830**	**36**
· with contact	484,810	1
· without contact	11,726,020	35
Household Crime	**14,817,360**	**44**
· Burglary	4,757,420	14
· Household larceny	8,101,150	24
· Motor vehicle theft	1,958,780	6

Source: Bureau of Justice Statistics

Violence, continued

Exhibit 26 (continued) Crime victimization: Total number by major category (in thousands)

Category	1973	1975	1980	1985	1990	1991	1992
Personal crimes	20,322	21,867	21,430	19,297	18,984	17,472	18,832
Household crimes	15,340	17,400	18,822	15,567	15,420	16,025	14,817

Source: Bureau of Justice Statistics

Costs of disease and injury

Exhibit 27. **Average annual cost of treating a person with AIDS, 1992**

Component of care	Medical care cost in 1992 dollars
Inpatient hospital	$22,680
Outpatient visits (clinic or office)	4,560
Long-term care	660
Home health care	2,088
Drugs	3,180
Outpatient subtotal	10,488
Total	$33,168

Source: Fred J. Hellinger, Forecasts of the Costs of Medical Care for Persons with HIV: 1992-1995, *Inquiry* 29 (Fall 1992): 356-365.
Fred J. Hellinger, The Lifetime Cost of Treating a Person with HIV, *JAMA*, July, 1993.

Exhibit 28. **Disease stage and lifetime treatment costs of AIDS, in 1992 dollars**

Disease stage	Mean occupancy time (months)	Cost per month	Total cost of care during stage
HIV-positive without AIDS (T-cel count >0.50x10^9/L)	67.3	$ 282	$18,978
HIV-positive without AIDS (T-cel count >0.20 and <0.50x10^9/L)	44.0	430	18,920
HIV-positive without AIDS (T-cel count <0.20x10^9/L)	12.4	990	12,276
With AIDS	25.0	2,764	69,100
Total lifetime care	148.7	802	119,274

Source: Fred J. Hellinger, The Lifetime Cost of Treating a Person with HIV, *JAMA*, July, 1993.

Costs of disease and injury, continued

Exhibit 29. **Cost of firearm Injuries by type of cost and class of injury (in millions of dollars)**

1985	*All*	*Fatal*	*Hospitalized*	*Non-hospitalized*
Total cost	$14,410	$12,172	$2,160	$78
· Direct	912	92	784	36
· Morbidity	1,418	–	1,376	43
· Mortality	12,080	12,080	–	–
1990				
Total cost	20,417	17,502	2,806	109
· Direct	1,410	141	1,209	60
· Morbidity	1,647	–	1,597	50
· Mortality	17,361	17,361	–	–

Source: Max and Rice, *Health Affairs,* Winter 1993

Exhibit 30. **Summary of victim injury costs per physical injury, in 1989 dollars**

Cost category	Rape and other injury	Robbery	Assault	Arson	Murder
Total monetary	**$6,228**	**$3,075**	**$2,991**	**$12,885**	**$ 671,136**
· Medical	1,367	430	678	1,490	6,467
· Emergency services	66	34	25	147	520
· Productivity	4,683	2,562	2,084	11,612	656,192
· Administrative	112	49	204	108	7,957
Total mental health	**36,306**	**10,387**	**5,802**	**1,224**	–
· Mental health medical	4,990	1,072	490	100	–
· Mental health productivity	1,465	333	202	48	–
· Quality of life lost to psychological injury	29,851	8,982	5,110	1,076	–
Quality of life	**17,842**	**11,485**	**13,521**	**35,022**	**1,715,918**
Total cost	**60,376**	**24,947**	**22,314**	**49,603**	**2,387,054**

Excludes property damage, legal costs, and employer costs. Includes rapes and attempted rapes that resulted in physical injury.
Source: Miller, Cohen and Rossman, *Health Affairs,* Winter 1993, pp.187-197

Costs of disease and injury

Exhibit 31. Lifetime costs of criminal victimizations, based on average annual incidence from 1987 to 1990, in millions of 1989 dollars

Cost category	Rape and other injury	Robbery	Assault	Arson	Murder	Total
Total monetary	**$483**	**$1,652**	**$7,894**	**$200**	**$13,564**	**$23,793**
· Medical	104	228	1,769	22	131	2,254
· Emergency services	12	39	155	2	11	219
· Productivity	358	1,359	5,438	174	13,261	20,590
· Administrative	9	26	532	2	161	730
Total mental health	**8,294**	**15,349**	**52,853**	**127**	**–**	**76,623**
· Mental health medical	1,140	1,586	4,464	10	–	7,200
· Mental health productivity	335	493	1,840	5	–	2,673
· Quality of life lost to psychological injury	6,819	13,270	46,549	112	–	66,750
Quality of life	**1,364**	**6,090**	**35,279**	**526**	**34,677**	**77,936**
Total cost	**10,141**	**23,091**	**96,026**	**853**	**48,241**	**178,352**

Excludes property damage, legal costs, and employer costs. Includes rapes and attempted rapes that resulted in physical injury.
Source: Miller, Cohen and Rossman, *Health Affairs,* Winter 1993

Health care delivery

Medical practice and health workforce

Physician-population ratios

Exhibit 32. **Number of physicians per 100,000 total population, 1950-1993**

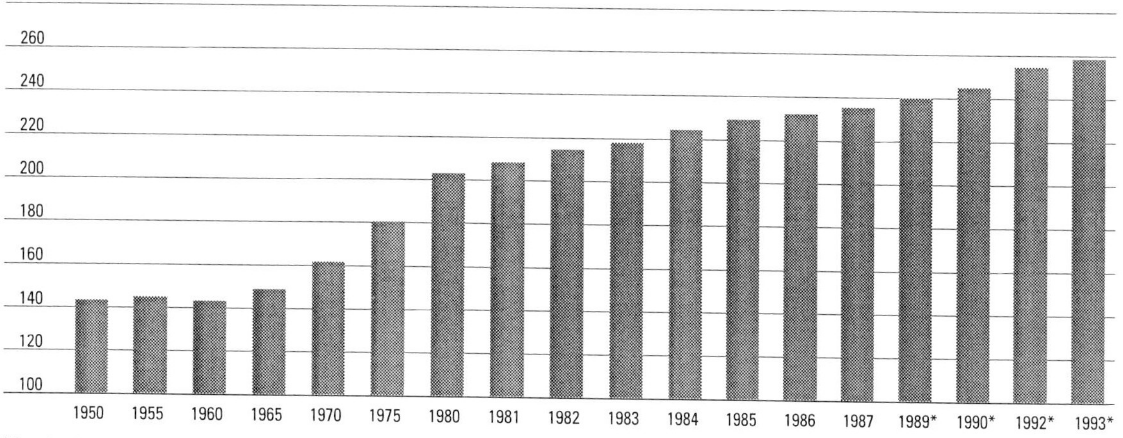

* Data for 1989, 1990, 1992 and 1993 are as of January 1. Data prior to 1989 are as of December 31.

Source: American Medical Association

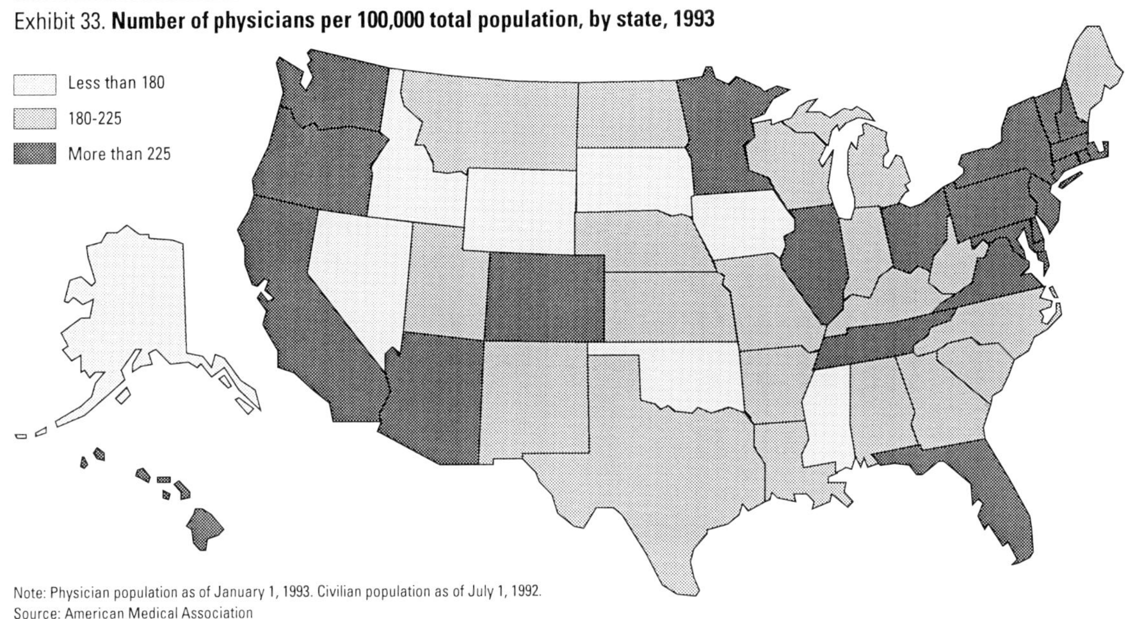

Note: Physician population as of January 1, 1993. Civilian population as of July 1, 1992.
Source: American Medical Association

Physicians: Supply, demographics and projections

Exhibit 34. **Physician population, by major activity and specialty**

Federal and non-federal physicians

	1970	1975	1980	1985	1990*	1992*	1993*
Total physician population	334,028	393,742	467,679	552,716	615,421	653,062	670,336
Federal	35,283	39,182	28,378	30,401	30,500	29,784	31,121
Non-federal	298,745	354,560	439,301	522,315	584,921	623,278	639,215
Total active population**	311,203	340,280	414,916	497,140	547,310	579,108	591,017

Major professional activity

	1970	1975	1980	1985	1990*	1992*	1993*
Total patient care	278,535	311,937	376,512	448,820	503,870	535,220	550,448
Office-based practice	192,439	215,429	272,000	330,197	360,995	389,364	398,854
Hospital-based practice							
· Residents	51,228	57,802	62,042	75,411	83,389	86,468	87,051
· Clinical fellows	—	—	—	—	8,691	7,128	6,579
· Hospital staff	34,868	38,706	42,470	43,212	50,795	52,260	57,964

Other professional activity

	1970	1975	1980	1985	1990*	1992*	1993*
Medical teaching	5,588	6,445	7,942	7,832	8,090	7,983	7,870
Administration	12,158	11,161	12,209	13,810	14,819	14,923	14,524
Research+	11,929	7,944	15,377	23,268	16,930	16,367	14,716
Other	2,635	2,793	2,876	3,410	3,601	3,615	3,459

Specialty

General/family practice***	57,948	54,557	60,049	67,051	70,480	71,688	71,685
Medical specialties	77,214	95,087	125,755	159,567	180,628	197,052	201,641
Surgical specialties	86,042	96,015	110,778	128,156	136,687	141,382	141,846
Other specialties	89,999	94,621	118,334	142,366	159,515	167,808	175,845
Not classified****	0	26,145	20,629	13,950	12,678	16,589	14,668
Inactive	19,621	21,449	25,744	38,646	52,653	55,656	62,997
Address unknown	3,204	5,868	6,390	2,980	2,780	2,709	1,654

* Data as of January 1. Data prior to 1990 are as of December 31.

**Total active physician population is the number of physicians who are classified and with a known address.

***Data on family practice were not available before 1975.

****Not classified was established in 1970; complete data were not available until 1972.

+ Includes physicians in research activities and research fellows.

Source: American Medical Association

Physicians: Supply, demographics and projections

Exhibit 35. **Physician population: Demographics**

Physician population by selected demographic features

	1970	1975	1980	1985	1990	1991	1993
Total physicians*	330,824	393,742	467,679	552,716	615,421	653,062	670,336
Gender distribution							
· % male	92.3	90.9	88.4	85.4	83.1	81.9	81.2
· % female	7.7	9.1	11.6	14.6	16.9	18.1	18.8
Age distribution							
· % under 35	26.7	27.5	27.5	25.6	21.9	20.5	20.0
· % 35-44	25.2	24.5	25.4	28.0	30.0	30.4	30.1
· % 45-54	21.4	20.9	18.8	18.0	19.0	19.7	20.3
· % 55-64	15.2	14.2	14.6	14.3	13.6	13.4	13.3
· % 65 and over	11.5	13.0	13.7	14.1	15.5	16.0	16.2
Median age of physicians*	46.0	46.1	46.2	46.3	47.1	47.4	47.6
IMG physicians	57,217	80,848	97,726	118,875	131,764	144,399	149,525
USMG physicians	273,607	312,894	369,953	433,841	483,657	508,663	520,811
*Location of Practice**							
· Metropolitan	85.7	87.1	86.9	86.6	88.1	88.4	88.5
· Non-metropolitan	14.3	12.9	13.1	13.4	11.9	11.6	11.5

*Excludes 3,204 physicians with unknown addresses.
**Excludes all physicians with unknown addresses.
Source: American Medical Association

Number and projected number of active physicians

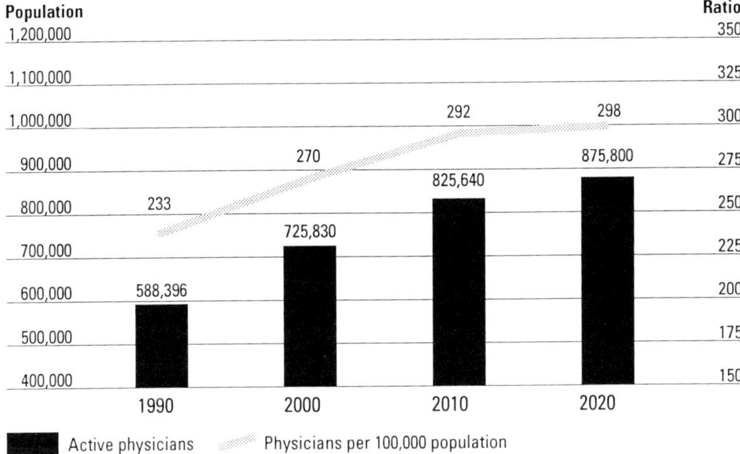

Source: American Medical Association

Medical education

Exhibit 37. **Undergraduate medical school application acceptancess**

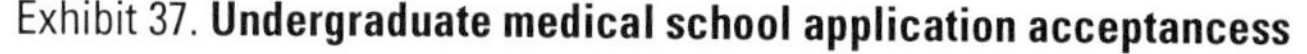

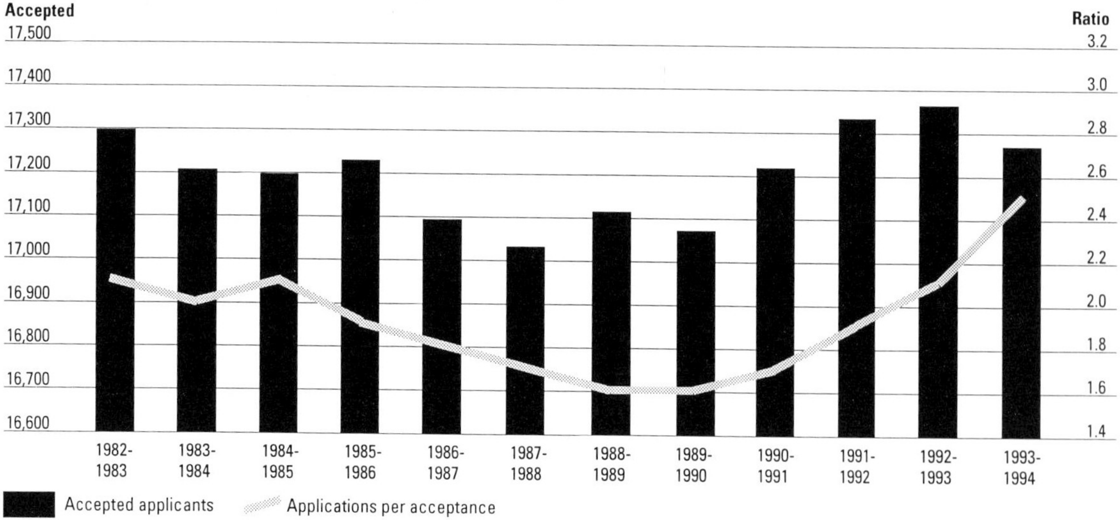

Souce: American Medical Association

Exhibit 38. **Undergraduate medical school, applicants, graduates, and enrollment**

	1985-1986	1986-1987	1987-1988	1988-1989	1989-1990	1990-1991	1991-1992	1992-1993	1993-1994
Applicants	32,893	31,323	28,123	26,721	26,915	29,243	33,301	37,410	42,808
First-year enrollment	16,929	16,779	16,686	16,781	16,749	16,803*	17,027	17,001	17,090
Percent female	34.2%	35.0%	36.5%	37.0%	38.2%	38.7%	39.8%	41.8%	42.2%
Medical school graduates	16,125	15,836	15,887	15,620	15,336	15,481	15,386	15,512	15,620+
Percent female	30.8%	32.1%	33.7%	33.5%	33.9%	36.1%	35.7%	38.1%	38.0%+
Total enrollment	66,604	66,142	65,742	65,150	65,081	64,986	65,539	65,969	66,453+
Percent female	32.5%	33.4%	34.3%	35.1%	36.1%	37.2%	38.0%	39.3%	40.2%+

* Meharry Medical College of Nashville, Tennessee did not provide first-year enrollment data. 1992-93 figures were used for this school.

+ Estimated in April 1991.

Source: *Journal of the American Medical Association*

Medical education, continued

Exhibit 39. **First-year medical students, by race**

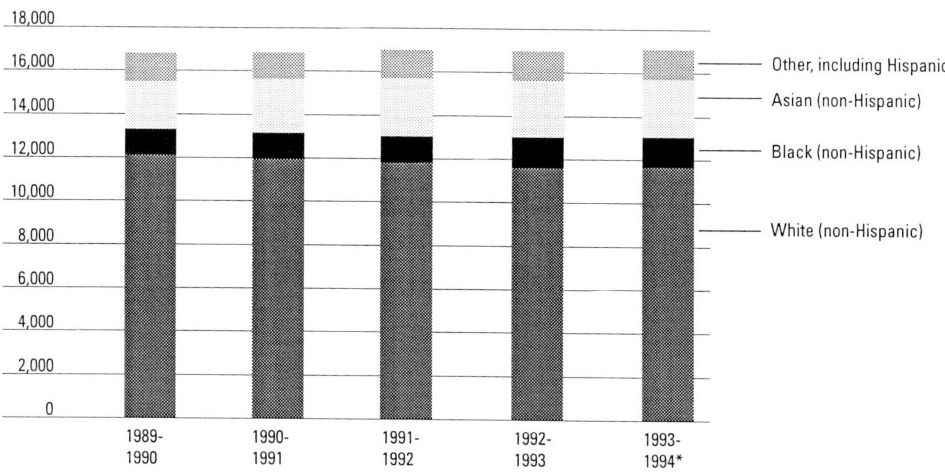

* Meharry Medical College of Nashville, Tennessee did not provide first-year enrollment data. 1992-93 figures were used for this school.

Source: *Journal of the American Medical Association*

Exhibit 40. Graduate medical school enrollment, by gender and place of graduation, by academic years

	1985-1986	1986-1987	1987-1988	1988-1989	1989-1990+	1990-1991	1991-1992	1992-1993	1993-1994
Total residents	74,514	76,815	81,410	81,093	85,330	82,902	86,217	89,368	97,370
By gender									
Female	19,562	20,746	22,623	21,879	23,673	24,492	25,923	27,760	31,198
Percent of total	26.3	27.0	27.8	27.0	27.7	29.5	30.1	31.1	32.0
Male	54,952	56,069	58,787	59,214	61,657	58,410	59,812	61,155	65,763
Percent of total	73.7	73.0	72.3	73.0	72.3	70.5	69.4	68.4	67.5
By place of graduation									
USMG	62,005	64,780	68,698	68,660	73,071	67,988	68,938	70,104	74,664
Percent of total	83.2	84.3	84.4	84.7	85.6	82.0	80.0	78.4	76.7
IMG	12,509	12,035	12,712	12,433	12,259	14,914	17,279	19,264	22,706
Percent of total	16.8	15.7	15.6	15.3	14.4	18.0	20.0	21.6	23.3
USIMG	6,868	5,845	5,822	5,131	4,814	5,026	5,107	5,015	5,056
Percent of total	9.2	7.6	7.2	6.3	5.6	6.1	5.9	5.6	5.2
Alien IMG	5,641	6,190	6,890	7,302	7,445	9,888	12,172	14,249	17,650
Percent of total	7.6	8.1	8.4	9.0	8.7	11.9	14.1	15.9	18.1

* Residents on duty September 1 of the academic year.
+ Projected.
Source: *Journal of the American Medical Association*

Medical education, continued

Exhibit 41. **Medical school expenditures, by function (in millions)**

	1980-1981		1985-1986		1990-1991		1991-1992	
Total expenditures	$ 6,366	100.0%	$ 10,817	100.0%	$ 20,370	100.0%	$ 22,445	100.0%
Instruction and research	2,386	37.5	3,865	35.7	6,060	29.7	6,293	28.0
Research	1,478	23.2	2,553	23.6	4,641	22.8	5,141	22.9
Service	708	11.1	1,283	11.9	4,169	20.5	5,048	22.5
Program support	797	12.5	1,313	12.1	2,241	11.0	2,429	10.8
Scholarships and fellowships	67	1.1	141	1.3	223	1.1	257	1.1
House staff	247	3.9	480	4.4	1,041	5.1	1,144	5.1
O and M of physical plant	357	5.6	542	5.0	748	3.7	805	3.6
Other functions	326	5.1	640	5.9	1,247	6.1	1,328	5.9

Data prepared by the Association of American Medical Colleges using the Liaison Committee on Medical Education questionnaires. Transfers are not included.

Source: *Journal of the American Medical Association*

Exhibit 42. **Sources of loans and scholarship funds**

	Millions of constant (1991) dollars			
	1981-82	*1990-91*	*1991-92*	*1992-93*
School-based financial assistance				
Total financial assistance	697	861	930	984
Total scholarships	216	194	213	221
Total loans	479	664	714	759
National programs and loans				
Scholarships				
· Armed Forces health professions	67	58	56	50
· National health servicec corps	58	1	5	7
· School funds	41	80	93	101
Loans				
· Stafford loan program	343	332	336	331
· Health education assistance and other alternative loans	50	145	169	196

Source: *Journal of the American Medical Association*

Medical education, continued

Exhibit 43. **Medical education indebtedness, by specialty certification group, 1992**

	Median debt	Percentage with no debt
Private schools		
Generalist specialties	$70,000	12.2%
Medical specialties	64,000	19.8
Surgical specialties	65,500	23.9
Support specialties	70,000	19.1
Total	**68,000**	**20.1**
Public schools		
Generalist specialties	45,000	16.1
Medical specialties	45,000	20.4
Surgical specialties	46,000	19.9
Support specialties	46,000	18.1
Total	**45,000**	**18.9**
All groups	50,000	19.4

Source: *Academic Medicine*

Exhibit 44. **Trends in productivity measures, all physicians**

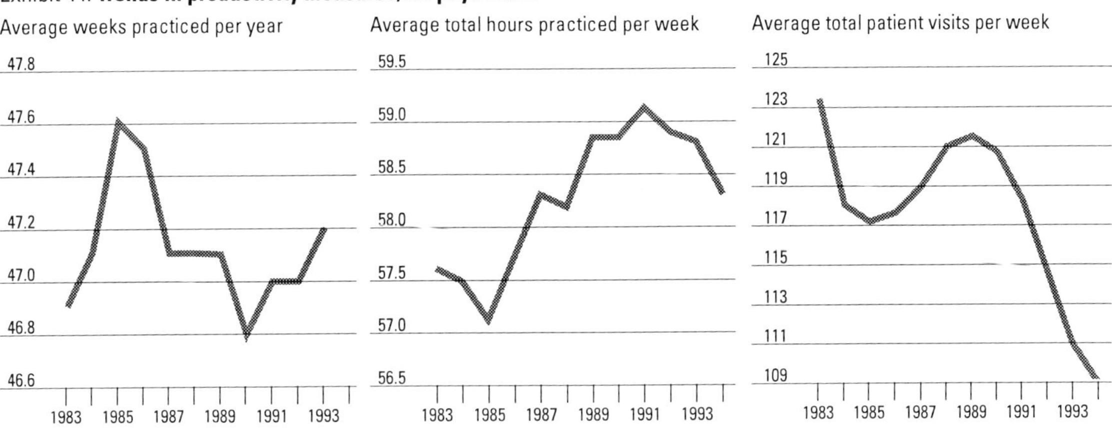

Source: American Medical Association

Physician productivity, continued

Exhibit 45. **Average weeks practiced per year, by specialty and employment status**

	1985	*1986*	*1987*	*1988*	*1989*	*1990*	*1991*	*1992*	*1993*
All	47.6	47.5	47.1	47.1	47.1	46.8	47.0	47.0	47.2
Specialty									
General/family practice	48.5	48.3	47.7	47.9	48.1	47.3	47.7	47.9	47.7
Medical specialties	47.9	47.9	47.4	47.3	47.2	47.2	47.4	47.5	47.5
Surgical specialties	47.5	47.2	47.0	47.0	47.0	46.6	46.7	46.8	47.4
Other	47.0	47.0	46.4	46.6	46.6	46.5	46.4	46.4	46.6
Employment status									
Self employed	47.6	47.6	47.5	47.4	47.5	47.3	47.4	47.7	47.7
Employed	47.3	47.2	46.0	46.4	46.2	45.6	46.1	45.8	46.6
Other (contractor)	–	–	–	–	–	46.7	46.5	45.7	46.6

Source: American Medical Association

Exhibit 46. **Average total practice hours per week, by specialty and employment status**

	1985	1986	1987	1988	1989	1990	1991	1992	1993	1994
All	57.1	57.7	58.3	58.2	58.8	58.8	59.1	58.9	58.8	58.3
Specialty										
General/family practice	58.6	57.9	58.2	58.3	58.8	59.7	60.1	58.5	59.1	56.5
Medical specialties	58.1	59.6	60.9	60.4	61.4	60.3	60.8	61.3	61.9	61.9
Surgical specialties	58.0	59.3	58.9	60.2	59.9	60.1	60.1	60.4	60.8	60.5
Other	54.3	54.3	55.5	53.8	55.1	55.6	55.8	54.8	53.4	53.4
Employment status										
Self employed	57.8	58.8	59.8	59.5	60.4	60.5	61.3	60.7	61.1	60.4
Employed	53.7	54.5	54.5	54.8	54.9	55.2	53.9	54.9	54.8	56.0
Other (contractor)	–	–	–	–	–	–	56.7	55.9	52.6	52.6

Source: American Medical Association

Physician productivity, continued

Exhibit 47. **Average total visits per week, by specialty and employment status**

	1985	1986	1987	1988	1989	1990	1991	1992	1993	1994
All	117.1	117.7	119.3	121.1	121.6	120.9	118.4	114.8	112.4	109.6
Specialty										
General/family practice	138.1	139.2	138.3	145.6	143.0	146.0	144.4	138.4	137.0	133.5
Medical specialties	111.9	116.7	117.7	118.6	123.0	117.4	116.4	116.7	111.7	110.5
Surgical specialties	109.2	108.0	109.0	108.5	109.7	110.6	108.2	103.9	101.5	99.9
Other	118.0	111.8	121.3	123.5	117.4	121.1	112.8	113.5	110.8	100.0
Employment status										
Self employed	123.2	121.3	123.2	124.7	126.2	126.4	124.1	119.2	118.0	117.0
Employed	102.5	106.8	107.8	110.6	109.1	107.3	102.5	101.4	100.2	98.2
Other (contractor)	–	–	–	–	–	–	117.7	124.2	112.2	105.3

Source: American Medical Association

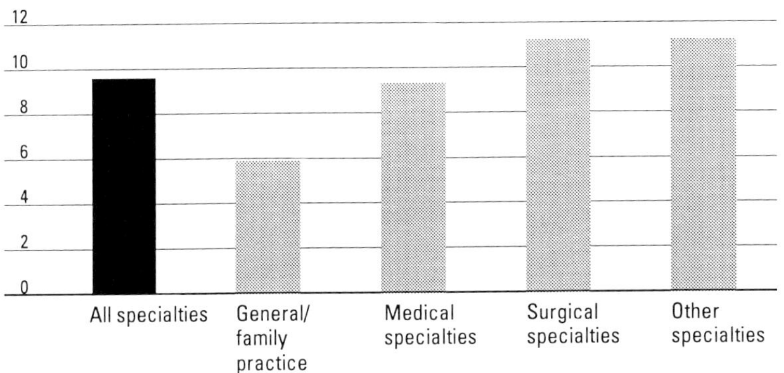

Excludes physicians in radiology, psychiatry, anesthesiology, and pathology.
Source: American Medical Association

Physician productivity, continued

Exhibit 49. **Waiting time for physicians, 1983-1994**

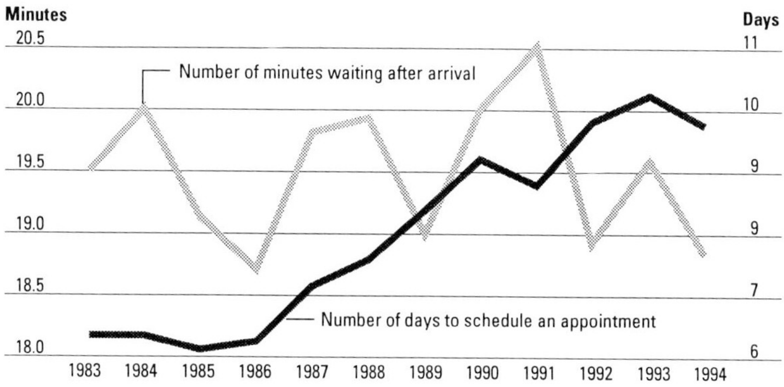

Excludes physicians in radiology, psychiatry, anesthesiology, and pathology.
Source: American Medical Association

Exhibit 50. **Total physician encounters with patients, 1995**

Estimated number per day (millions)

	NHIS	*SMS*
Patient visits*	5.5	7.6
Base encounters+	5.7	7.8
Add: Admissions and discharges	5.9	8.0
Add: Telephone calls	6.4	9.0
Add: Adjustment for surgery	6.5	9.1

NHIS is the National Health Information Survey, a patient-based survey.

SMS is the Socioeconomic Monitoring System, a physician-based survey.

* Office visits, inpatient hospital visits, and visits in outpatient settings.

+ Patient visits, surgical procedures, and hospital diagnostic and nonsurgical procedures.

Source: American Medical Association

Physician income and expenses

Exhibit 51. **Average physician income and expenses, annual percentage change**

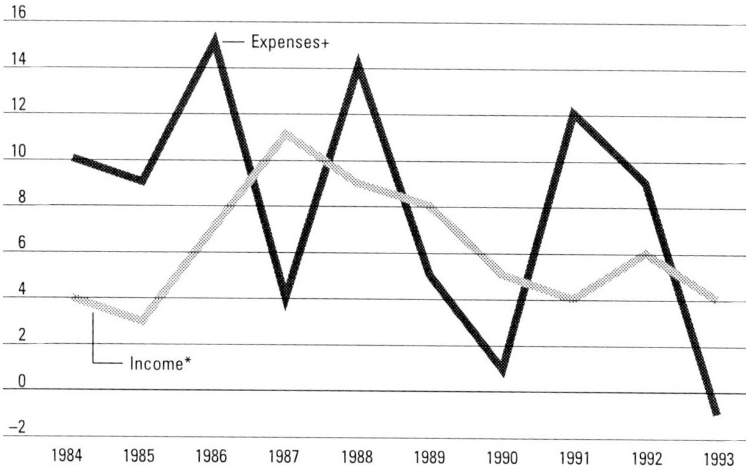

* After expenses but before taxes.
+ For self-employed physicians.
Source: American Medical Association

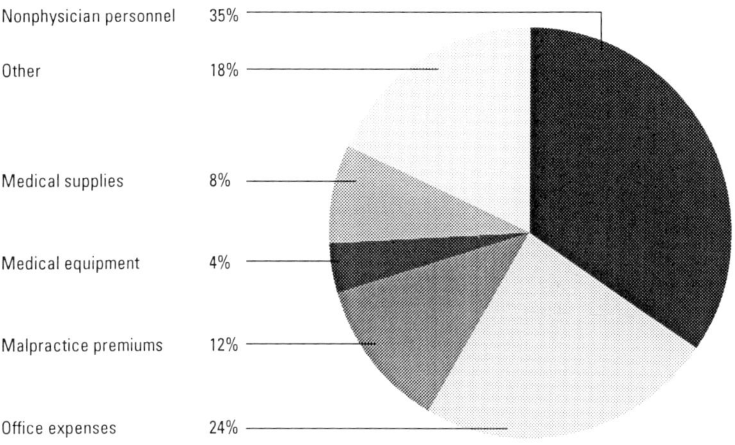

* Based on responses from self-employed physicians who provided necessary information. Components may not add to 100% because of rounding.
Source: American Medical Association

Physician income and expenses, continued

Exhibit 53. **Average professional expenses (in thousands) of self-employed physicians, by specialty**

	1985	*1986*	*1987*	*1988*	*1989*	*1990*	*1991*	*1992*	*1993*
All	$102.7	$118.4	$123.7	$140.8	$148.4	$150.0	$168.4	$183.4	$182.2
Specialty									
General/family practice	96.5	119.9	121.2	122.3	128.5	134.5	146.4	162.9	162.4
Medical specialties	89.3	106.6	113.8	131.6	137.6	138.9	156.1	174.0	181.7
Surgical specialties	134.8	148.8	166.9	188.5	202.0	203.2	220.4	243.8	244.0
Other	81.0	92.1	80.4	100.7	101.5	103.2	122.3	126.7	114.2

Source: American Medical Association

Exhibit 54. **Average net income (in thousands), by specialty, age and employment status**

	1985	*1986*	*1987*	*1988*	*1989*	*1990*	*1991*	*1992*	*1993*
All	$112.2	$119.5	$132.3	$144.7	$155.8	$164.3	$170.6	$181.7	$189.3
Specialty									
General/family practice	77.9	80.3	91.5	94.6	95.9	102.7	111.5	114.4	116.8
Medical specialties	94.8	102.2	112.3	121.3	136.0	140.4	142.1	152.5	169.5
Surgical specialties	147.6	156.1	181.8	200.2	214.0	229.0	230.6	242.8	251.9
Other	113.9	125.0	132.6	145.5	154.9	163.0	177.4	188.8	188.6
Age									
Less than 36 years	88.3	95.9	100.2	112.2	119.7	123.6	134.9	132.2	143.6
Less than 40	98.1	105.9	117.1	130.9	137.9	148.8	157.2	163.0	169.9
36-45	119.1	125.9	141.0	157.5	165.2	173.6	179.1	192.5	196.3
46-55	131.2	138.8	152.9	162.0	181.0	191.9	188.7	208.0	214.0
56-65	110.0	118.3	128.3	137.2	150.4	160.8	169.4	180.9	194.3
66 or over	86.4	79.1	93.9	98.8	105.9	100.8	114.1	120.3	120.0
Employment status									
Self-employed	124.5	131.1	146.2	160.0	175.3	185.6	191.0	202.3	218.0
Employee	83.8	91.7	99.6	113.0	119.2	119.8	129.3	136.1	150.7
Other (contractor)	—	—	—	—	—	147.6	157.1	138.6	159.9

* Net income is after expenses and before taxes.
Source: American Medical Association

Liability and malpractice

Exhibit 55. Average professional liability claims per 100 physicians, by specialty

	1985	1986	1987	1988	1989	1990	1991	1992	1993
All	10.2	9.2	6.7	6.4	7.4	7.7	8.2	9.1	9.8
Specialty									
General/familypractice	5.7	7.6	5.7	6.2	6.6	5.9	5.7	6.9	7.1
Medicalspecialties	6.4	5.8	4.5	4.2	5.8	7.1	5.7	7.3	6.9
Surgicalspecialties	19	15.2	11.5	11.4	11.8	11.6	13.4	15.5	19.8
Other	8	7.8	4.9	4.1	5.2	5.5	7.4	6.4	5.4

Source: American Medical Association

Exhibit 56. Average professional liability premiums (in thousands) per self-employed physician, by specialty

	1985	1986	1987	1988	1989	1990	1991	1992	1993
All*	$10.5	$12.8	$15.0	$15.9	$15.5	$14.5	$14.9	$13.8	$14.4
Specialty									
General/family practice	6.8	7.3	8.9	9.4	9.0	7.8	8.1	8.2	7.9
Internal medicine	5.8	7.1	8.4	9.0	8.2	9.2	8.0	8.6	9.0
Surgery	16.6	21.3	24.5	26.5	25.8	22.8	22.5	20.9	22.7
Pediatrics	4.7	6.3	7.1	9.3	7.8	7.8	8.4	7.7	8.6
Obstetrics/gynecology	23.5	29.3	35.3	35.3	37.0	34.3	34.9	34.0	33.7

*Includes specialties not listed separately.
Source: American Medical Association

Exhibit 57. **Change in average professional liability insurance premiums for self-employed physicians by specialty, 1984-85 to 1992-93**

(Annual percentage change from previous year)

	1985	*1986*	*1987*	*1988*	*1989*	*1990*	*1991*	*1992*	*1993*
All*	25.2%	21.9%	17.2%	6.0%	−2.5%	−6.5%	2.8%	−7.4%	4.3%
Specialty									
General/family practice	47.1	7.4	21.9	5.6	−4.3	−13.3	3.8	1.2	−3.7
Internal medicine	19.3	22.4	18.3	7.1	−8.9	12.2	−13.0	7.5	4.7
Surgery	24.8	28.3	15.0	8.2	−2.6	−11.6	−1.3	−7.1	8.6
Pediatrics	37.2	34.0	12.7	31.0	−16.1	0.0	7.7	−8.3	11.7
Obstetrics/gynecology	23.9	24.7	20.5	0.0	4.8	−7.3	1.7	−2.6	−0.9

*Includes specialties not listed separately.
Source: American Medical Association

Liability and malpractice, continued

Exhibit 58. **Ten most frequent malpractice allegations, 1994**

Allegation	Number	Average cost
1. Surgery/postoperative complications	996	$61,828
2. Failure to diagnose/cancer	490	108,811
3. Surgery/inadvertent act	398	77,672
4. Improper treatment/birth related	370	178,349
5. Failure to diagnose/fracture or dislocation	210	60,417
6. Improper treatment/drug side effect	203	71,826
7. Failure to diagnosis/abdominal problems/other	168	89,467
8. Improper treatment/infection	168	72,958
9. Failure to diagnose/myocardial infarction	132	130,803
10. Improper treatment/fracture or dislocation	126	52,995

Source: *Physicians' & Surgeons' Update*

Exhibit 59. **Ten most costly malpractice allegations, by average cost, 1994**

Allegation	*Number*	*Average cost**
1. Improper treatment/birth related	370	$178,349
2. Failure to diagnose/hemorrhage	65	134,557
3. Failure to diagnose/myocardial infarction	132	130,803
4. Failure to diagnose/infection	165	113,120
5. Failure to diagnose/cancer	490	108,811
6. Failure to diagnose/circulatory problem/thrombosis	177	106,258
7. Surgery/post-operative death	127	103,177
8. Failure to diagnose/pregnancy problems	85	101,436
9. Failure to diagnose/abdominal problems	168	89,467
10. Surgery/inadvertant act	398	77,672

*The average cost includes the total value of claim including allocated legal expenses with no cap on individual claims.
Based on the average cost of loss allegations in 10 claims or more.

Source: *Physicians' & Surgeons' Update*

Liability and malpractice, continued

Exhibit 60. Median and average medical malpractice verdict awards

Year	Median	Average
1984	$200,000	$ 640,619
1985	400,000	1,179,095
1986	355,000	1,216,195
1987	318,000	911,413
1988	300,000	908,686
1989	348,607	1,202,109
1990	433,000	1,650,798
1991	440,000	1,424,615
1992	365,107	1,761,747
1993	500,000	1,964,816
1994	392,790	1,342,493

* Data are incomplete.

Source: Copyright 1995 by LRP Publications, 747 Dresher Road, Horsham, PA 19044-0980. For more information on Jury Verdict Research Publications published by LRP Publications, please call 800 341-7874, ext. 233

Exhibit 61. Underwriting premiums and losses for the medical malpractice insurance industry (in billions)

Year	Net premiums written	Dollar losses incurred and loss adjustment expense
1978	$1.22	$1.05
1980	1.28	1.37
1982	1.49	1.82
1984	1.77	2.47
1986	3.49	4.14
1988	4.03	4.13
1989	4.28	3.09
1990	4.02	3.44
1991	4.07	3.33
1992	4.13	4.36
1993	4.37	3.37
1994	4.78	3.58

Source: *Best's Aggregates and Averages*

Exhibit 62. **Number of active osteopathic physicians relative to the total physician population**

	1986	1990	Projected		
			2000	2010	2020
Physician population					
All physicians	544,830	601,060	721,600	810,160	848,620
MDs	522,020	573,310	682,182	759,630	789,560
DOs	22,810	27,750	39,480	50,530	59,060
Rate per 100,000 US population					
All physicians	224.9	240.0	269.0	286.7	288.3
MDs	215.5	228.9	254.3	268.8	268.2
DOs	9.4	11.1	14.7	17.9	20.1
Percent distribution					
All physicians	100.0	100.0	100.0	100.0	100.0
MDs	95.8	95.4	94.5	93.8	93.0
DOs	4.2	4.6	5.5	6.2	7.0

Source: US Department of Health and Human Services

Health care workforce

Exhibit 63. **Active health personnel and their number per 100,000 population, by occupation**

	1970	1980	1990	1991
Number of health personnel				
Physicians[a]	290,862	409,480	546,827	579,822
· Doctors of Medicine[b]	279,212	393,407	520,451[c]	551,932
· Doctors of Osteopathy	11,650	16,073	26,376	27,890
Dentists[d]	95,700	121,240	145,500	158,600
Optometrists	18,400	22,330	26,000	26,500
Pharmacists	112,570	142,780	161,900	163,600
Podiatrists	7,110	8,880	12,000	12,500
Registered nurses	750,000	1,272,900	1,715,600	1,758,500
· Associate and diploma	–	908,300	1,077,800	1,100,400
· Baccalaureate	–	297,300	517,800	533,500
· Masters and doctorate	–	67,300	120,000	124,700
Veterinarians	25,900	36,000	51,000	52,400

Number per 100,000 population[e]

Physicians[a]	142.7	182.0	221.8	231.4
· Doctors of Medicine[b]	137.0	174.9	211.1[c]	220.3
· Doctors of Osteopathy	5.7	7.1	10.7	11.1
Dentists[d]	47.0	53.5	58.4	63.3
Optometrists	9.0	9.8	10.4	10.4
Pharmacists	55.4	62.5	64.4	64.4
Podiatrists	3.5	4.0	4.8	4.9
Registered nurses	368.9	560.0	690.0	697.3
· Associate and diploma	–	399.9	433.4	436.4
· Baccalaureate	–	130.9	208.2	122.6
· Masters and Doctorate	–	29.6	48.3	49.4
Veterinarians	12.7	16.3	20.4	20.6

a Non-federal.
b Excludes physicians not classified according to activity status.
c Doctors of Medicine data are reported as of January 1. Doctors of Osteopathy are reported as of December 31.
d Excludes dentists in military service.
e Ratios for physicians and dentists are based on civilian population ratios for all other health occupations are based on resident population.
Source: US Department of Health and Human Services

Health care workforce, continued

Exhibit 64. **Graduates of health professions schools, by profession**

	1970	1975	1980	1985	1990	1991	1992*	2000+
Medicine	8,367	12,714	15,135	16,319	15,336	15,481	15,466	16,536
Osteopathy	432	702	1,059	1,474	1,529	1,533	1,537	1,758
Nursing#	43,103	73,915	75,523	82,075	66,088	72,230	80,839	61,800
Dentistry	3,749	4,969	5,256	5,353	4,233	3,995	3,918	3,242
Optometry	445	806	1,073	1,114	1,115	1,136	1,150	1,200
Pharmacy	4,758	6,712	7,278	5,724	6,956	7,122	–	7,120
Chiropractic	642	1,093	2,049	–	–	–	–	2,950

* Data for medicine are estimated.

+ Projected.

Registered nurses only.

Source: US Department of Health and Human Services

Exhibit 65. **Employment in selected medical-related industries**

	Average employment (in thousands) July of:		
	1991	*1993**	*Change*
Health services	8,218.8	8,920.1	8.5%
Offices/clinics of medical doctors	1,407.7	1,555.1	10.5
Offices/clinics of dentists	528.2	564.7	6.9
Offices/clinics—other health practitioners	303.5	356.4	17.4
Nursing and personal care facilities	1,506.7	1,620.7	7.6
· Skilled nursing care facilities	1,079.6	1,154.7	6.9
· Intermediate care facilities	212.1	231.9	9.3
· Nursing and personal care	215.0	234.1	8.9
Hospitals	3,672.3	3,838.8	4.5
· General medical and surgical hospitals	3,375.5	3,530.6	4.6
· Psychiatric hospitals	104.7	100.3	−4.2
· Specialty hospitals, excluding psychiatric	192.1	207.9	8.2
Medical and dental laboratories	173.6	194.7	12.2
Home health care services	345.3	478.5	38.6

* Preliminary.
Source: US Department of Labor

Health care delivery

Hospitals

Hospital utilization

Exhibit 66. **Total number of beds, admissions, and outpatient visits (in thousands)**

Year	Beds	Admissions	Outpatient visits
1950	1,456	18,483	—
1955	1,604	21,073	—
1960	1,658	25,027	—
1965	1,704	28,812	125,793
1970	1,616	31,759	181,370
1975	1,466	36,157	254,844
1980	1,365	38,892	262,951
1985	1,318	36,304	282,140
1990	1,213	33,774	368,184
1991	1,202	33,567	387,675
1992	1,178	33,536	417,874
1993	1,163	33,201	435,619

Source: *AHA Hospital Statistics*, 1994/95 edition. Copyright by the American Hospital Association

Exhibit 67. **Growth in the numbers of hospital beds, admissions and outpatient visits**

Average annual percent change

Year	Beds	Admissions	Outpatient visits
1950-55	2.0%	2.7%	–
1955-60	0.7	3.5	–
1960-65	0.5	2.9	–
1965-70	−1.1	2.0	7.6%
1970-75	−1.9	2.6	7.0
1975-80	−1.4	1.5	0.6
1980-85	−0.7	−1.2	1.4
1985-90	−1.6	−1.6	5.5
1990-93	−1.4	−0.6	5.8

Source: *AHA Hospital Statistics,* 1994/95 edition. Copyright by the American Hospital Association

Hospital utilization, continued

Exhibit 68. **Annual percentage changes in hospital utilization measures**

Period	Beds	Admissions	Outpatient visits
1980-1981	−0.2%	0.7%	0.9%
1981-1982	−0.1	−0.2	18.2
1982-1983	−0.7	−0.5	−12.9
1983-1984	−0.8	−2.4	1.2
1984-1985	−1.6	−4.3	2.0
1985-1986	−2.1	−3.0	4.4
1986-1987	−1.8	−2.2	5.5
1987-1988	−1.5	−1.0	8.2
1988-1989	−1.8	−1.1	4.8
1989-1990	−1.1	0.1	4.5
1990-1991	−0.9	−0.6	5.3
1991-1992	−2.0	−0.1	7.8
1992-1993	−1.3	−1.0	4.2

Source: *AHA Hospital Statistics,* 1994/95 edition. Copyright by the American Hospital Association

Exhibit 69. **Average length of stay in community hospitals by ownership type (in days)**

Year	All	Private not-for-profit*	For-profit	State/local government
1972	7.9	8.0	6.6	8.0
1975	7.7	7.8	6.6	7.6
1980	7.6	7.7	6.5	7.3
1985	7.1	7.2	6.1	7.2
1990	7.2	7.3	6.4	7.7
1991	7.2	7.2	6.3	7.8
1992	7.1	7.1	6.3	7.9
1993	7.0	6.9	6.2	7.8

*Excludes government community hospitals.

Source: *AHA Hospital Statistics,* 1994/95 edition. Copyright by the American Hospital Association

Hospital utilization, continued

Exhibit 70. **Registered hospital units by defining characteristics**

	1972	1982	1993	Change 72-82	Change 82-93
Total facilities	6338	6933	6467	9.4%	−6.7%
By size					
6-24 beds	382	305	290	−20.2%	−4.9%
25-49	1370	1150	1065	−16.1%	−7.4%
50-99	1618	1674	1554	3.5%	−7.2%
100-199	1321	1597	1582	20.9%	−0.9%
200-299	673	806	834	19.8%	3.5%
300-399	393	502	471	27.7%	−6.2%
400-499	238	333	253	39.9%	−24.0%
500 or more	343	566	418	65.0%	−26.1%
Federal	341	348	316	2.1%	−9.2%
· Psychiatric	2	24	19	1100.0%	−20.8%
· General/other	339	324	297	−4.4%	−8.3%
Non-federal	5997	6585	6151	9.8%	−6.6%
Total community	5746	5813	5261	1.2%	−9.5%

By Location

New England	269	252	227	−6.3%	−9.9%
Middle Atlantic	656	615	561	−6.3%	−8.8%
South Atlantic	748	823	790	10.0%	−4.0%
E-N Central	893	904	809	1.2%	−10.5%
E-S Central	467	492	449	5.4%	−8.7%
W-N Central	781	797	714	2.0%	−10.4%
W-S Central	825	847	743	2.7%	−12.3%
Mountain	357	367	350	2.8%	−4.6%
Pacific	750	716	618	−4.5%	−13.7%

Source: *AHA Hospital Statistics,* 1972, 1982, and 1994/95 editions. Copyright by the American Hospital Association

For-profit and multihospital systems

Exhibit 71. **Number of for-profit hospitals and beds, total and as a percentage of total for community hospitals**

Year	For-profit hospitals total number	Percent of total hospitals	For-profit beds total number*	Percent of total beds
1972	738	12.8%	57	6.5%
1975	775	13.2	73	7.7
1980	730	12.5	87	8.8
1985	805	14.0	104	10.4
1990	749	13.9	101	10.9
1991	738	11.1	100	8.3
1992	723	11.0	99	8.4
1993	717	11.1	99	8.5

*In thousands.

Source: *AHA Hospital Statistics,* 1994/95 edition. Copyright by the American Hospital Association

 Growth in the number of beds at for-profit and non-profit community hospitals

(percentage change from previous year)

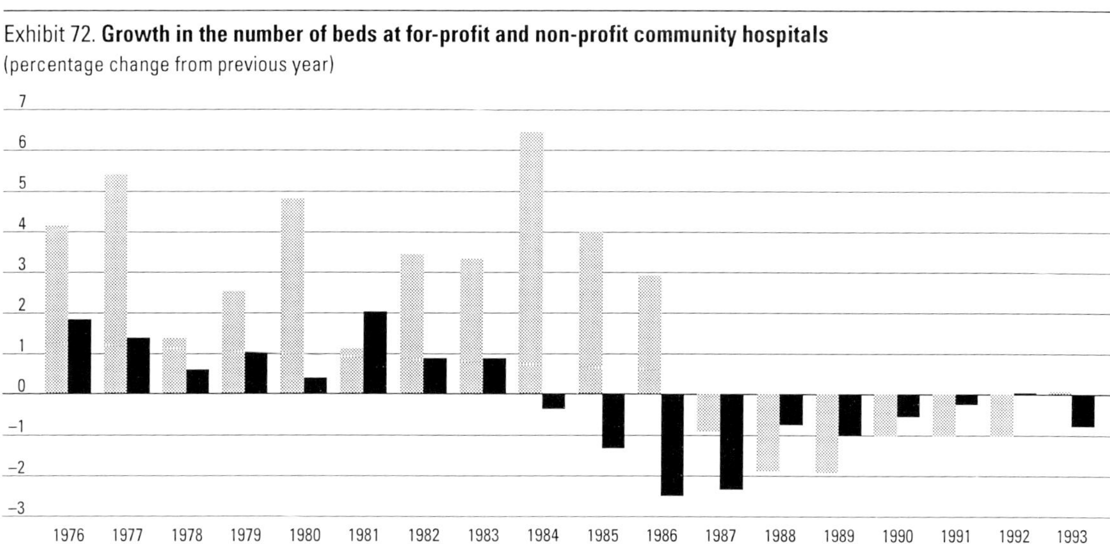

*Excludes government community hospitals.

Source: *AHA Hospital Statistics,* 1994/95 edition. Copyright by the American Hospital Association

For-profit and multihospital systems, continued

Exhibit 73. **Annual growth in the number of beds at community hospitals by ownership and multihospital system status**

		Ownership status		Multihospital system status	
Year	All hospitals	For-profit	Not-for-profit*	Member	Independent
1985	−1.6	4.0	−1.3	8.2	−8.7
1986	−2.3	2.9	−2.5	0.1	−4.3
1987	−2.0	−0.9	−2.3	1.3	−6.4
1988	−1.1	−1.9	−0.7	0.7	−2.6
1989	−1.5	−1.9	−1.0	21.6	−21.4
1990	−0.6	−1.0	−0.6	4.8	−7.5
1991	−0.3	−1.0	−0.2	−1.8	1.4
1992	−0.3	−1.0	0.0	−1.6	1.6
1993	−0.2	0.0	−0.8	na	na

*Excludes government community hospitals.
na—not available.
Source: *AHA Hospital Statistics,* 1994/95 edition; *AHA Guide to the Health Care Field,* 1991, 1992, and 1993 editions. Copyright by the American Hospital Association

Year	Total hospitals	% of total hospitals	Total beds	% of total beds
1979	1,797	30.8%	341,382	34.7%
1982	1,958	33.8	365,914	36.2
1985	2,476	43.2	429,367	42.9
1986	2,514	44.3	429,837	44.0
1987	2,567	45.7	435,422	45.5
1988	2,572	46.5	438,433	46.3
1989	2,901	53.2	533,290	57.2
1990	2,906	54.0	558,664	60.3
1991	2,873	53.8	548,759	59.4
1992	2,826	53.4	540,099	58.6

Source: *AHA Guide to the Health Care Field,* 1983-1993 editions. Copyright by the American Hospital Association

Unsponsored and uncompensated care

Exhibit 75. **Unsponsored and uncompensated care as a percentage of costs, by type of hospital**

Hospital type	1980		1989	
	Uncompensated	Unsponsored	Uncompensated	Unsponsored
All hospitals	5.1%	3.6%	6.0%	4.8%
Urban	5.2	3.6	6.1	4.8
Rural	4.3	3.8	5.5	4.9
Major teaching	9.6	3.8	8.6	4.2
Other teaching	4.0	3.7	5.6	5.2
Non-teaching	3.9	3.4	5.2	4.8
Voluntary	3.6	3.5	5.0	4.9
Urban gov't	12.9	4.2	12.4	4.6
Rural gov't	5.1	3.8	6.7	4.8

Uncompensated care is the estimated cost of bad debt and charity care to the hospital.
Unsponsored care is equal to uncompensated care minus hospitals' revenues from state and local government tax appropriations.
Source: Congressional Budget Office

Exhibit 76. **Real uncompensated and unsponsored care provided by hospitals**

(Billions of 1991 dollars)

Year	Uncompensated	Unsponsored
1983	$8.3	$6.6
1984	9.7	7.3
1985	9.6	7.6
1986	11.1	8.6
1987	11.4	8.6
1988	12.0	9.3
1989	12.2	9.8
1990	12.6	9.9
1991	13.4	10.8

Uncompensated care is the estimated cost of bad debt and charity care to the hospital.

Unsponsored care is equal to uncompensated care minus hospitals' revenues from state and local government tax appropriations.

Source: Congressional Budget Office

International hospital comparisons

Exhibit 77. **Use of acute care hospitals and physicians in selected countries, 1990**

Country	Hospitalizations per 100 population	Physician contacts per capita
France	21.0	7.2
Austria	20.5	5.8
Germany	18.5	11.5
Belgium	17.0	7.6
Italy	16.8	11.0
Sweden	16.3	2.8
Switzerland	13.9	6.0
Canada	13.8	6.9
United Kingdom	12.9	5.7
United States	12.4	5.5
Netherlands	10.3	5.5
Japan	8.3	12.9

Source: American Medical Association

Exhibit 78. **Acute hospital beds and employees per bed in selected countries, 1990**

Country	Beds per 1,000 population	Employees per bed
Germany	7.5	1.3
Switzerland	6.5	1.9
Italy	6.4	1.4
Austria	6.0	0.9
Belgium	5.6	1.2
France	5.2	1.1
Canada	4.3	2.5
Netherlands	4.3	2.1
Sweden	3.9	3.4
United States	3.6	3.1
United Kingdom	2.8	2.6

Source: American Medical Association

Health care delivery

Managed care systems

Physician participation in managed care

Exhibit 79. **Percentage of physicians with managed care contracts**

	1990	1991	1992	1993	1994
Contract with any type of managed care provider	61%	65%	70%	75%	77%
Contract with					
IPA	19	20	21	26	32
HMO	36	37	42	48	55
PPO	49	54	58	66	65

Source: American Medical Association

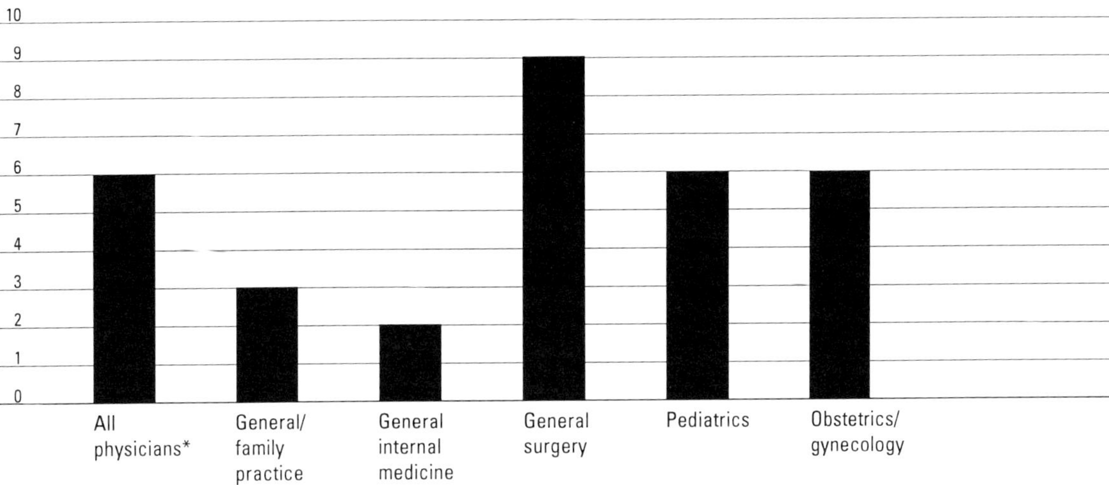

Note: *Includes specialties not listed separately.
Source: American Medical Association

Physician participation in managed care, continued

Exhibit 81. **Capitation and withholds, by specialty, 1994**

	Percent of revenue from managed care	Percent capitated	Percent with withholds
All physicians*	34%	15%	19%
Specialty			
General/family practice	34	22	22
General internal medicine	31	22	27
General surgery	36	10	14
Pediatrics	40	20	26
Obstetrics/gynecology	44	14	20

Note: *Includes specialties not listed separately.
Source: American Medical Association

Exhibit 82. **Distribution of operational PPOs by ownership category, 1993**

Ownership category	Number sponsored	Percent of total
Insurance carrier	347	45%
Independent investor	155	20
Physician-hospital joint venture	45	6
Hospital alliance	36	5
Physician medical group	32	4
Hospital	29	4
Third party administrator	21	3
Multi-ownership	21	3
HMOs	13	2
Employer-employer coalition	8	1
Others	57	7
Total	763	100%

Source: Marion Merrell Dow *Managed Care Digest, PPO Edition 1994* and SMG Marketing Group

HMOs and PPOs, continued

Exhibit 83. **Growth of HMOs**

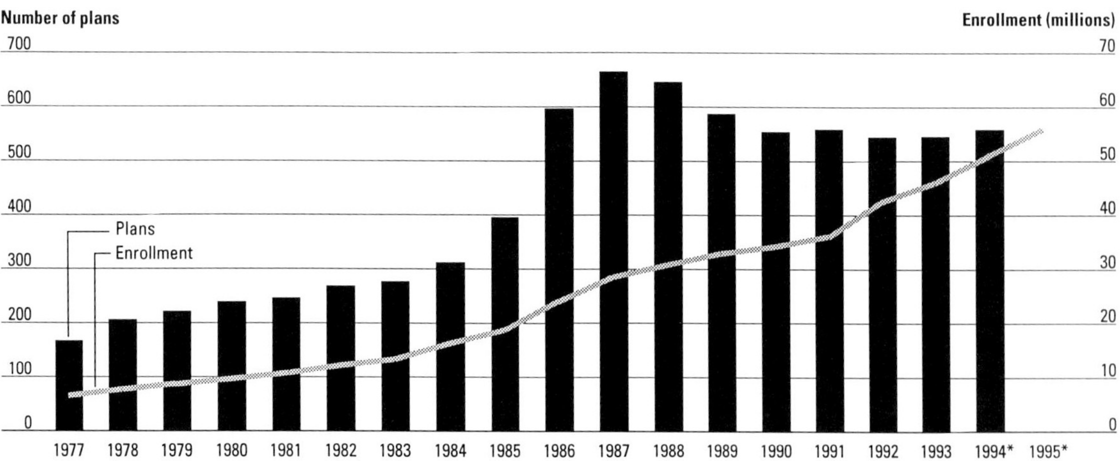

Note: All numbers are as of June 30 or July 1 of a year, except 1992, which is as of December 1, and 1993, which is a year-end figure, and 1994 which is as of March 1.
*Estimate.

Sources: *Managed Care Outlook,* Capitol Publications Inc., PO Box 1453, Alexandria, VA 22313-2053, 703 683-4100; InterStudy; *Statistical Abstract of the United States*

Exhibit 84. **State penetration of HMOs, by year end 1993***

States with 25% or more penetration (high)

Arizona	32.9
California	35.0
District of Columbia	37.6
Massachusetts	34.1
Minnesota	30.1
Oregon	31.5
Rhode Island	25.9

States with 15-24% penetration (moderate)

Colorado	23.2
Connecticut	24.5
Delaware	17.2
Florida	17.6
Hawaii	22.3
Illinois	16.1
Michigan	18.4
New Mexico	15.7
New York	21.4
Ohio	15.2
Pennsylvania	18.9
Utah	18.5
Washington	15.2
Wisconsin	23.1

States with 5-14% penetration (low)

Alabama	6.4
Georgia	7.1
Indiana	6.7
Kansas	7.5
Kentucky	6.6
Louisiana	7.1
Missouri	14.3
Nebraska	6.7
Nevada	12.7
New Hampshire	13.6
New Jersey	13.0
North Carolina	6.6
Oklahoma	7.3
Tennessee	5.7
Texas	9.7
Vermont	11.1
Virginia	7.2

States with 0-4% penetration (negligible)

Alaska	0.0
Arkansas	2.8
Idaho	1.1
Iowa	3.8
Maine	4.3
Maryland	3.2
Mississippi	0.1
Montana	1.4
North Dakota	0.5
South Carolina	3.3
South Dakota	2.9
West Virginia	0.0
Wyoming	0.0

*Penetration is defined as the percentage of state population with health insurance enrolled in an HMO.

Source: *Managed Care Outlook,* Capitol Publications Inc., PO Box 1453, Alexandria, VA 22313-2053, 703 683-4100

Managed care in the health insurance market

Exhibit 85. **Managed care market share**

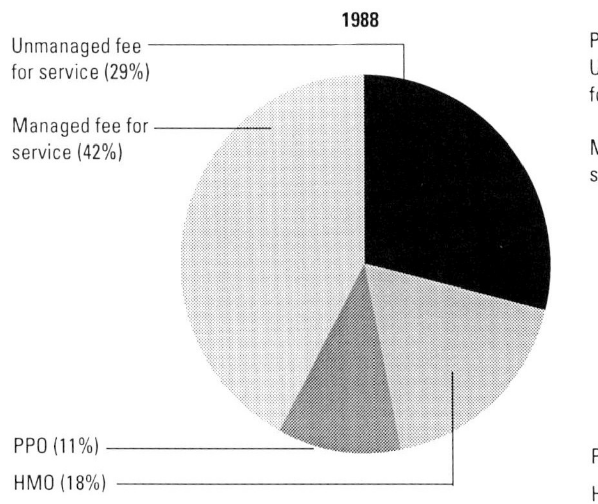

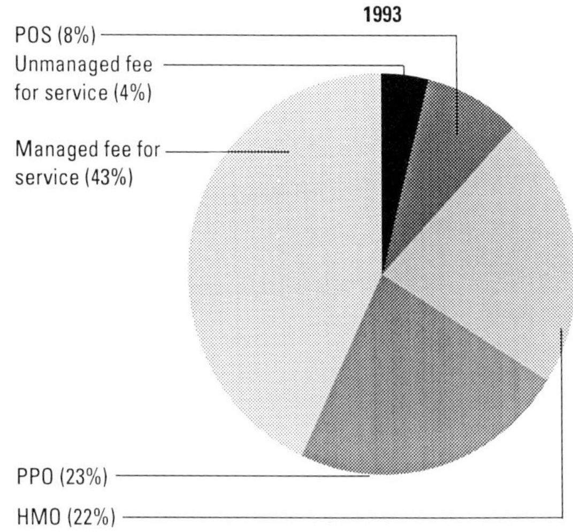

Source: American Medical Association

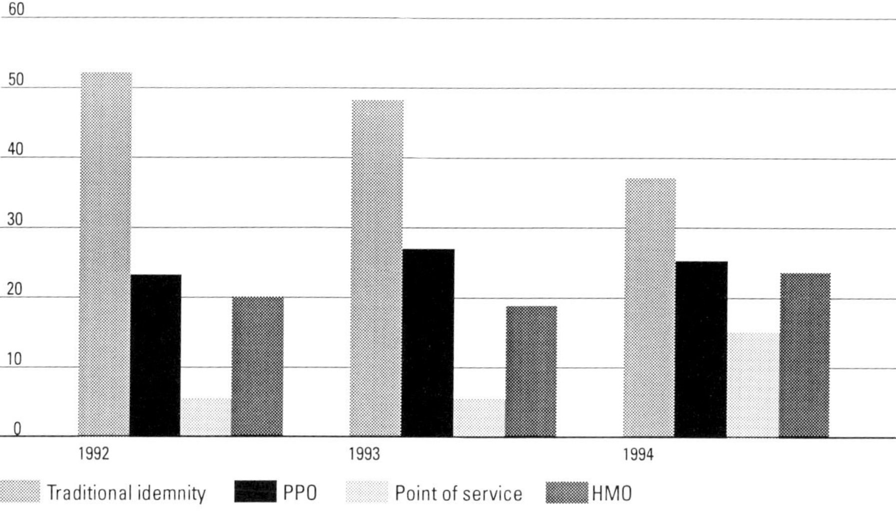

Source: Foster Higgins

Managed care in the health insurance market, continued

Exhibit 87. **Average monthly health insurance premium cost, 1995**

	Individual coverage	*Family coverage*
Indemnity	$199	$544
HMO	153	432
PPO	173	474
POS	182	486

Source: *Managed Care Outlook,* Capitol Publications Inc., PO Box 1453, Alexandria, VA 22313-2053, 703 683-4100

Exhibit 88. **Growth in health insurance premiums**

	Percent change from previous year			
	1991	*1992*	*1993*	*1994*
All plan types	11.5%	10.9%	8.0%	4.8%
Traditional indemnity	12.0	11.0	8.5	5.1
PPO	10.1	10.6	8.2	3.2
POS	12.4	4.9	5.9	na
HMO	12.1	9.8	8.3	5.3

na = not available
Source: KPMG Peat Marwick LLP

Health care financing

National health expenditures

Exhibit 89. **National health expenditures as a percentage of GDP**

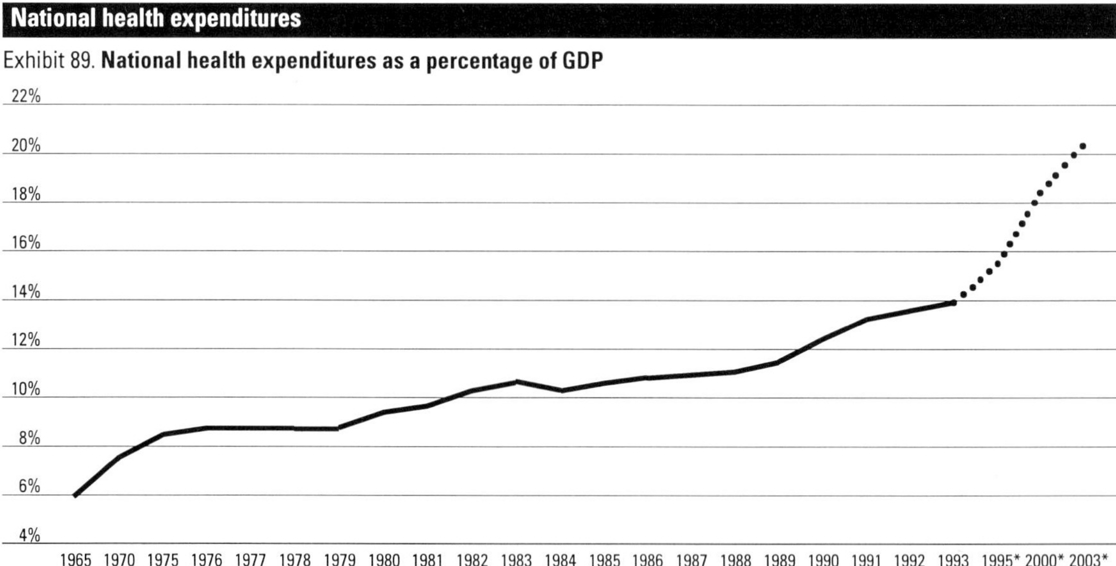

* Projected by CBO.

Source: Health Care Financing Administration; Congressional Budget Office

Where it came from

Private health insurance (32%)

Government programs (13%)

Medicaid (13%)

Medicare (19%)

Other private sources (5%)

Out-of-pocket payments (18%)

Where it went

Hospital care (37%)

Other spending (12%)

Other personal health care (24%)

Physician services (19%)

Nursing home care (8%)

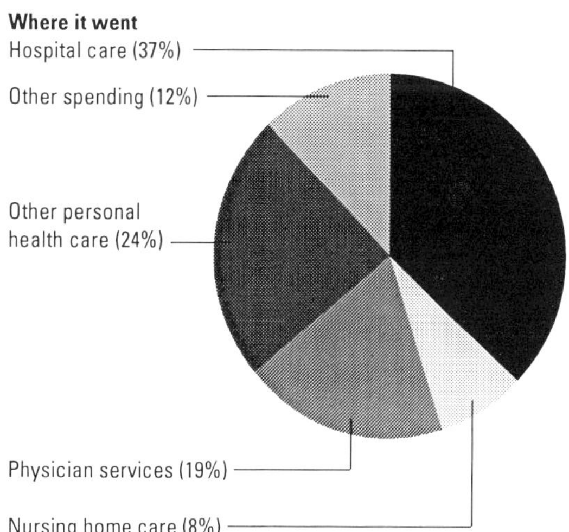

Source: Health Care Financing Administration

National health expenditures, continued

Exhibit 91. **Distribution of personal health care expenditures, by source of funds (percentage of total)**

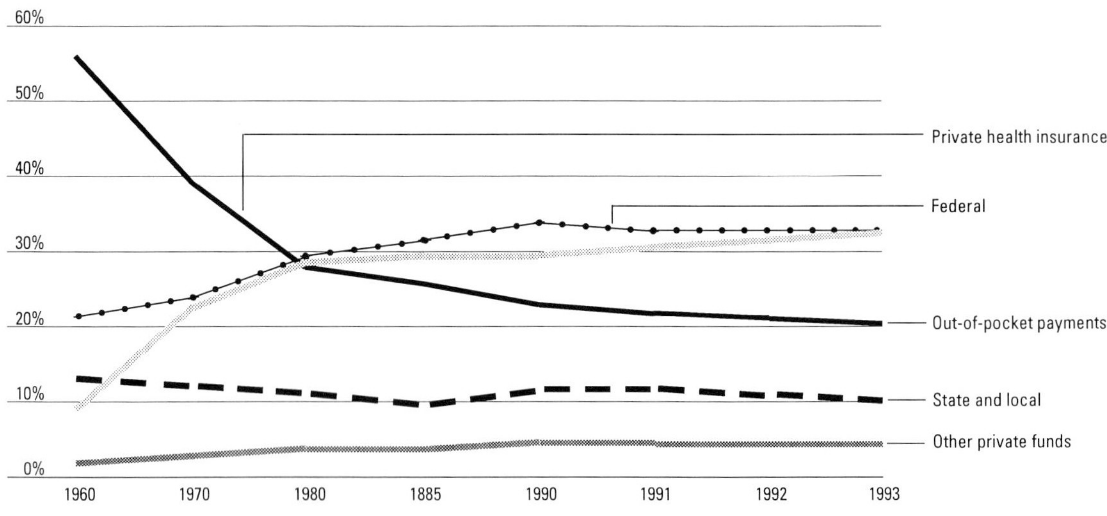

Source: Health Care Financing Administration

Year	Total NHE (in billions)	Average annual percent increase from previous year shown	Percent of GDP
1960	$27.1	–	5.3%
1970	74.3	10.6%	7.4
1980	251.1	12.9	9.3
1985	434.5	11.6	10.8
1987	506.2	7.9	11.1
1989	623.9	11.0	11.9
1990	696.6	11.6	12.6
1991	755.6	8.5	13.2
1992	820.3	8.6	13.6
1993	884.2	7.8	13.9

Source: Health Care Financing Administration

National health expenditures, continued

Exhibit 93. **Regional differences in health care expenditures, 1991**

Region	Expenditures per capita*	As a percent of US average
New England	$2,112	113%
Mideast	2,105	112
Plains	1,866	99
Far West	1,856	99
Great Lakes	1,826	97
Southeast	1,825	97
Southwest	1,705	91
Rocky Mountain	1,567	83
United States, overall	$1,877	100%

*Expenditures include hospital care, physician services, and retail purchases of prescription drugs.
Source: *Statistical Bulletin*

Exhibit 94. **National health expenditures, by type of expenditure (in billions of dollars)**

	1970	*1980*	*1990*	*1991*	*1992*	*1993*
National health expenditures	$74.3	$251.1	$696.6	$755.6	$820.3	$884.2
All health services and supplies	69.0	239.4	672.2	730.8	792.9	855.2
Personal health care	64.8	220.1	612.4	670.8	729.7	782.5
· Hospital care	28.0	102.7	256.5	282.3	306.0	326.6
· Physicians services	13.6	45.2	140.5	150.3	161.8	171.2
· Dental services	4.7	13.3	30.4	31.7	34.7	37.4
· Other professional services	1.4	6.4	36.0	40.4	46.4	51.2
· Home health care	0.2	1.9	11.1	13.2	16.8	20.8
· Medical products	10.8	26.1	71.7	78.4	82.8	87.6
· Nursing home care	4.9	20.5	54.8	60.8	65.5	69.6
· Other personal health care	1.3	4.0	11.4	13.8	15.8	18.2
Program administration and net cost of private health insurance	2.8	12.1	38.3	37.0	39.5	48.0
Government public health activities	1.4	7.2	21.6	22.9	23.7	24.7
Research and construction	5.3	11.6	24.3	24.8	27.4	29.0
Research*	2.0	5.5	12.2	12.9	14.2	14.4
Construction	3.4	6.2	12.1	11.9	13.2	14.6

* Research and development expenditures of drug companies and other manufacturers and providers of medical equipment and supplies are excluded form "research expenditures," but they are included in the expenditure class in which the product falls.

Source: Health Care Financing Administration

National health expenditures, continued

Exhibit 95. **Projections of national health expenditures (in billions of dollars)**

	1995	*2000*	*2003*
Total expenditures	$1,069	$1,613	$2,052
Gross domestic product	6,951	8,857	10,169
Expenditures as a % of GDP	15.4%	18.2%	20.2%
By type of spending			
Hospital	400	604	778
Physician	204	315	401
Drugs, other nondurables	80	112	137
Nursing home	91	138	176
All other	294	444	560
By source of funds			
Private	568	824	1,022
Public, federal	346	555	735
Public, state and local	156	234	295

Source: Congressional Budget Office

Country	Millions of US$	Per capita (US$)	As a percent of GDP	Public share of total	Private share of total
Established market economies, overall	$1,483,285	$1,958	9.29%	61.1%	38.9%
Australia	22,736	1,294	7.67	69.6	30.4
Austria	13,193	1,711	8.38	66.4	33.6
Belgium	14,428	1,449	7.50	82.5	17.5
Canada	51,594	1,945	9.05	74.1	25.9
Denmark	8,160	1,588	6.30	84.2	15.8
Finland	10,200	2,046	7.82	83.3	16.7
France	105,467	1,869	9.40	74.2	25.8
Germany	120,072	1,511	8.73	72.7	27.3
Greece	3,609	359	5.39	76.0	24.0
Iceland	480	1,884	8.34	87.5	12.5
Ireland	3,068	876	7.22	81.1	18.9
Italy	82,214	1,655	7.54	77.7	22.3
Japan	187,930	1,538	6.45	74.5	25.5
Luxembourg	628	1,662	6.56	91.4	8.6

(continued on next page)

Total health expenditures, selected countries, 1990, continued

Country	Millions of US$	Per capita (US$)	As a percent of GDP	Public share of total	Private share of total
Netherlands	$22,423	$1,501	8.03%	72.6%	27.4%
New Zealand	3,150	925	7.37	81.7	18.3
Norway	7,782	1,835	7.35	95.7	4.3
Portugal	3,970	383	6.99	61.7	38.3
Spain	3,275	831	6.59	78.4	21.6
Sweden	20,055	2,343	8.79	89.3	10.7
Switzerland	16,916	2,520	7.52	68.5	31.5
United Kingdom	59,623	1,039	6.11	84.9	15.1
United States	691,211	2,765	12.61	44.1	55.9

Source: World Health Organization

Exhibit 97. **Health insurance primary coverage enrollment**

	1980	*1990*	*1993*	*1995**	*2000**	*2003**
Employment-based insurance	148.0	153.1	148.6	149.2	152.2	154.0
Individual insurance	15.5	14.7	15.1	14.6	14.9	15.1
Medicare	24.0	30.5	32.6	33.7	35.5	36.2
Medicaid	11.5	14.6	20.5	22.6	26.4	27.7
Total population	223.2	246.2	254.2	259.1	270.1	276.2

*Projected.
Source: Congressional Budget Office

Medicare and Medicaid, continued

Exhibit 98. **Medicare and Medicaid public expenditures on personal health care**

Year	Medicare—Federal (in billions)	Medicaid (in billions)		
		Total*	Federal	State and local
1970	$7.6	$5.3	$2.9	$2.5
1980	37.5	26.1	14.5	11.6
1985	72.0	41.8	23.1	18.6
1986	76.9	45.2	25.4	19.8
1987	82.9	50.8	27.9	22.9
1988	90.5	54.9	31.0	23.9
1989	102.6	62.5	35.4	26.8
1990	110.7	75.5	42.8	32.7
1991	122.8	100.5	55.9	44.6
1992	135.4	103.4	65.9	37.7
1993	151.1	112.8	73.2	39.6

* May not add due to rounding.
Source: Health Care Financing Administration

Exhibit 99. **Number of Medicaid recipients, total payments, and average payment per recipient, by eligibility category, fiscal year 1992**

| | Medicaid recipients | | Medicaid payments | | |
| | *Number (thousands)* | *Percent distribution* | *Total amount (millions)* | *Percent distribution* | *Average payment per recipient* |
Eligibility category					
Total*	31,150	100.0%	$91,480	100.0%	$2,937
Aged > 65 years	3,749	12.0	29,089	31.8	7,759
Blindness	84	0.3	530	0.6	6,293
Permanent and total disability	4,402	14.1	33,474	36.6	7,604
Dependent children < 21 years	15,200	48.8	14,758	16.1	971
Adults in families with dependent children	7,040	22.6	12,403	13.6	1,762
Other categories of eligibility	675	2.2	1,226	1.3	1,817

* Categories do not add to total because of the small number of recipients that are in more than one eligibility category during the year.

Source: Social Security Administration

Medicare and Medicaid, continued

Exhibit 100. Medicare Part A and Part B per capita average reimbursement per aged and disabled person enrolled, by type of service and age, 1993

		Per capita Part A payments			Per capita Part B payments		
	Total all services	Inpatient hospital	Skilled nursing facility	Home health agency	Physician-related services	Outpatient	Home health agency
All aged enrollees	$3,519	$1,888	$129	$278	$1,004	$318	$4
By age group							
· 65-66	2,238	1,221	30	89	725	272	2
· 67-68	2,539	1,382	36	110	807	286	2
· 69-70	2,799	1,591	44	167	866	300	2
· 71-72	3,117	1,678	65	182	944	313	3
· 73-74	3,414	1,845	78	217	1,008	323	5
· 75-79	3,993	2,134	129	311	1,128	347	4
· 80-84	4,585	2,385	230	489	1,203	345	7
· >85	5,083	2,586	411	648	1,230	339	7

All disabled enrollees	4,123	2,228	45	192	1,065	773	0
By age group							
· < 35	4,115	2,332	19	102	947	871	0
· 35-44	3,794	2,048	30	146	959	795	0
· 45-54	3,898	2,046	41	165	1,039	777	0
· 55-59	4,320	2,312	58	230	1,144	767	0
· 60-64	4,564	2,483	73	273	1,217	688	0

Source: Health Care Financing Administration

Medicare and Medicaid, continued

Exhibit 101. **Medicare program enrollees and outlays (in millions)**

	Part A: Hospital insurance		Part B: Supplementary medical		Total, both programs**	
Year***	Number enrolled	Total outlays	Number enrolled	Total outlays	Number enrolled	Total outlays
1970	20,361	$4,953	19,584	$2,196	20,491	$7,149
1975	24,640	10,612	23,905	4,170	24,959	14,782
1980	28,067	24,288	27,400	10,737	28,478	35,025
1985	30,589	48,654	29,989	22,730	31,083	71,384
1990	33,731	66,687	32,636	43,022	34,213	109,709
1991	34,429	69,642	33,237	47,024	34,870	116,666
1992	35,159	81,971	33,956	50,285	35,598	132,256
1993	–	91,604	–	54,254	–	145,858
1994*	–	102,892	–	58,490	–	161,382
1995*	–	112,258	–	66,144	–	178,402
1996*	–	123,359	–	73,665	–	197,024
1997*	–	135,197	–	81,825	–	217,022
1998*	–	147,664	–	90,981	–	238,645
1999*	–	161,540	–	101,552	–	263,092

*HCFA Projection.

**Total Enrollees from Part A and Part B do not add to total Medicare enrollees because frequently one person will enroll in both programs.

***Enrollment as of July 1 and outlays are for fiscal years.

Source: Congressional Budget Office; Congressional Committee on Ways and Means; and the Health Care Financing Administration

Exhibit 102. **Medicaid total payments and payments per eligible recipient, by type of service, fiscal year 1993**

Type of service	Average total Medicaid amount (millions)	Percent distribution	Payment per recipient
All services*	$91,480	100%	$2,937
Inpatient services	25,886	28.3	32,551
Intermediate care facility services	8,552	9.3	56,517
Skilled nursing facility services	23,547	25.7	14,970
Physician services	6,122	6.7	282
Dental services	853	0.9	149
Other practitioner services	539	0.6	114
Outpatient hospital services	5,296	5.8	349
Clinic services	2,825	3.1	684
Laboratory and radiological services	1,040	1.1	88
Home health services	4,888	5.3	5,276
Prescribed drugs	6,790	7.4	308
Family planning services	504	0.6	197
Other care	4,637	5.1	366

* May not add due to rounding.
Source: Social Security Administration

Medicare and Medicaid, continued

Exhibit 103. **Medicare benefit payments (in billions) and annual percent change**

Calendar year	Part A: Hospital insurance	Part B: Supplementary medical insurance	Total benefit payments*	Average annual change from previous year shown
1966	$0.9	$0.1	$1.0	–
1970	5.1	2.0	7.1	7.5%
1975	11.3	4.3	15.6	25.5
1980	25.1	10.6	35.7	21.7
1981	30.3	13.1	43.5	21.7
1982	35.6	15.5	51.1	17.6
1983	39.3	18.1	57.4	12.4
1984	43.2	19.7	62.9	9.5
1985	47.6	22.9	70.5	12.1
1986	49.8	26.2	76.0	7.8
1987	49.5	30.8	80.3	5.7
1988	52.5	34.0	86.5	7.7
1989	60.0	38.3	98.3	13.7
1990	66.2	42.5	108.7	10.6
1991	71.5	47.2	118.7	9.2
1992	83.9	49.3	133.2	12.2

* May not add due to rounding.
Source: Social Security Administration

Exhibit 104. **Distribution of Medicare reimbursements for aged and disabled beneficiaries, by type of service, 1991**

Type of service	Amount reimbursed (millions) and type of beneficiary			Percent of total Medicare reimbursement
	Aged	*Disabled*	*Total*	
Hospital insurance	$61,474	$7,512	$68,986	62.2%
· Inpatient hospital	54,366	7,045	61,411	55.4
· Skilled nursing services	2,151	87	2,238	2.0
· Home health services	4,958	379	5,337	4.8
Supplementary Medical insurance	36,910	4,991	41,901	37.8
· Physician/other medical services	28,965	3,054	32,019	28.9
· Outpatient services	7,870	1,937	9,807	8.8
· Home health services	76	— *	76	0.1
Total	98,384	12,503	110,887	100.0

* Less than 500.
Source: Social Security Administration

Medicare and Medicaid, continued

Exhibit 105. **Distribution of enrollee costs under Medicare**

Cost category	1975	1980	1985	1990	1995*	2000*
Copayments	$117	$204	$363	$582	$790	$1,193
· HI copayments	34	66	117	188	246	329
· SMI copayments	83	138	246	394	544	864
Balance billing	22	56	87	68	42	67
Premium costs	80	110	186	343	553	728
Total enrollee costs	219	371	637	993	1,385	1,988

* Projected.
Source: Congressional Budget Office

Exhibit 106. **Percentage of Medicare enrollee costs, by category**

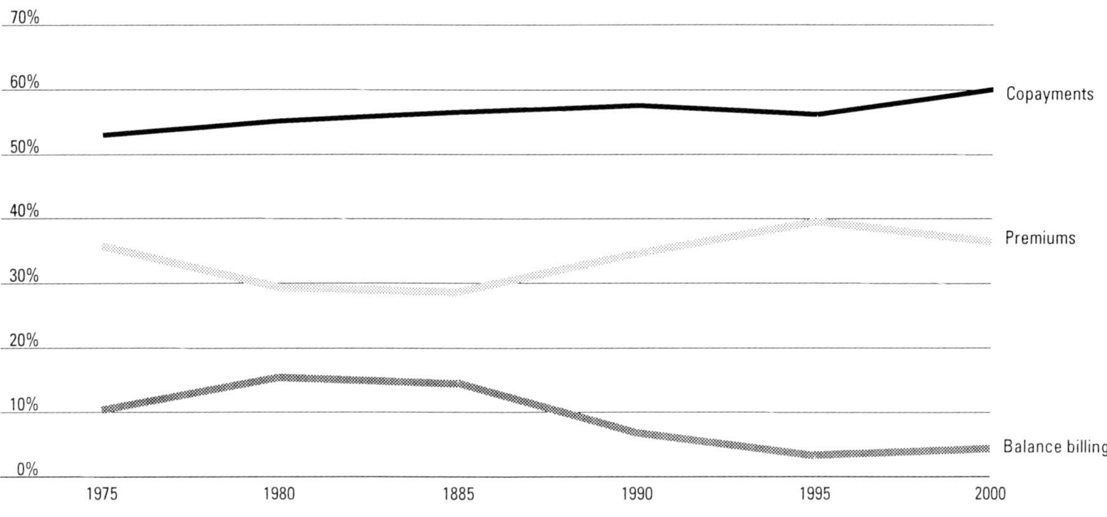

1995 and 2000 values are projected. All figures are in current dollars.
Source: Congressional Budget Office

Medicare and Medicaid, continued

Exhibit 107. **Medicare enrollment and payments, according to survival status**

	1976	1980	1985	1988
All Medicare beneficiaries (millions)	23.4	25.2	27.2	29.1
Number of beneficiaries who died during the year (millions)	1.22	1.35	1.45	1.49
Deceased as a percent of all beneficiaries	5.2%	5.4%	5.3%	5.1%
Total Medicare payments (billions)	$15.2	$31.0	$57.2	$73.0
Percent of total payments to deceased*	28.2%	30.8%	27.4%	28.6%

*Adjusted to 1976 values for age, sex and survival status of deceased.

Source: Adapted from JD Lubitz and GE Riley, *N Engl J Med,* 1993, Vol. 328, pp. 1092-96. Copyright 1993. Massachusetts Medical Society. All rights reserved.

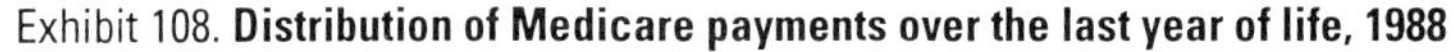
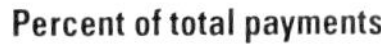

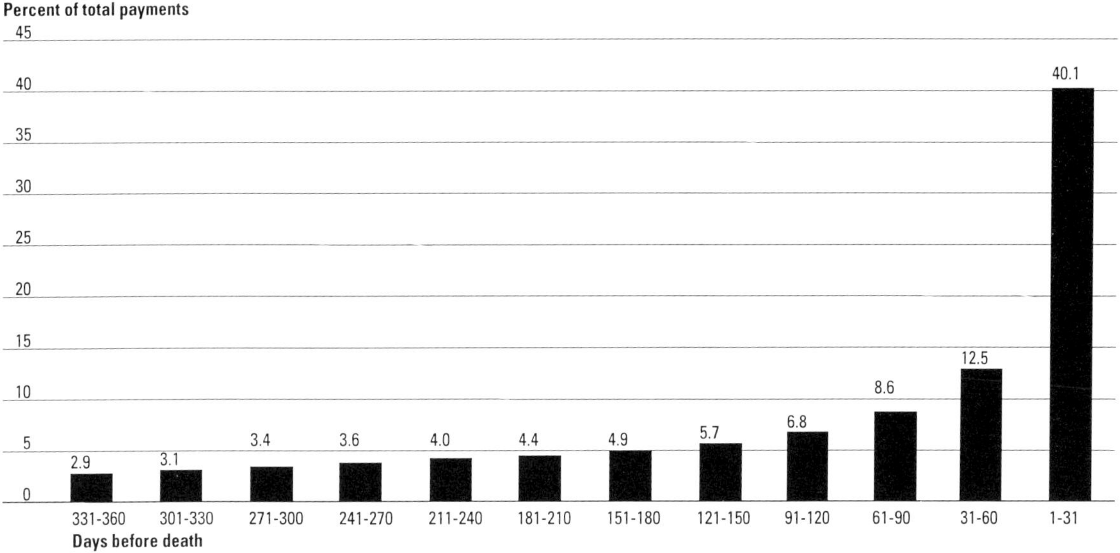

Source: Adapted from JD Lubitz and GE Riley, *N Engl J Med,* 1993, Vol. 328, pp. 1092-96. Copyright 1993. Massachusetts Medical Society. All rights reserved.

Private insurance

Exhibit 109. **Population under 65 years without health insurance, by selected characteristics, 1993**

Uninsured characteristics	Total population (in millions)	Number uninsured (in millions)	As a % total population in group	Percent of total uninsured
Total	226.2	40.9	18.1%	100.0%
Age				
Adult (18 years and older)	157.4	29.8	18.9	72.9
Children	68.8	11.1	16.1	27.1
Family income				
< $10,000	30.1	9.9	32.9	24.2
$10,000-19,999	32.6	10.8	33.1	26.4
$20,000-29,999	32.4	7.4	22.8	18.1
$30,000-39,999	29.4	4.6	15.6	11.2
> $40,000	101.6	8.2	8.1	20.0
Race				
Hispanic	25.0	8.5	34.0	20.8
White	162.9	23.7	14.5	57.9
Black	29.5	6.8	23.1	16.6
Other	8.7	1.9	21.8	4.6

Family income as a percentage of the poverty line				
0-99%	35.9	11.8	32.9	28.9
100%-149%	20.6	7.1	34.5	17.4
150%-199%	21.4	5.9	27.6	14.4
200% or more	148.3	16.0	10.8	39.1
Firm size of greatest earner				
Non-worker	27.0	6.3	23.3	15.4
Less than 10 employees	35.4	11.1	31.4	27.1
10-99 employees	43.4	9.9	22.8	24.2
100-499 employees	29.7	4.3	14.5	10.5
500 or more employees	90.6	9.3	10.3	22.7

Source: Employee Benefit Research Institute

Private insurance, continued

Exhibit 110. **Population under 65 years with health insurance, by selected characteristics, 1993**

Insured characteristics	Total population (in millions)	Number insured (in millions)	As a % total population in group	Percent of total insured
Total	226.2	185.3	81.9%	100%
Age				
Adult (18 years and older)	157.4	127.6	81.1	68.9
Children	68.8	57.7	83.9	31.1
Family income				
< $10,000	30.1	20.2	67.1	10.9
$10,000-19,999	32.6	21.8	66.9	11.8
$20,000-29,999	32.4	25.0	77.2	13.5
$30,000-39,999	29.4	24.8	84.4	13.4
> $40,000	101.6	93.4	91.9	50.4
Race				
Hispanic	25.0	16.5	66.0	8.9
White	162.9	139.2	85.5	75.1
Black	29.5	22.7	76.9	12.3
Other	8.7	6.8	78.2	3.7

Family income as a percentage of the poverty line				
0-99% of poverty	35.9	24.1	67.1	13.0
100%-149% of poverty	20.6	13.5	65.5	7.3
150%-199% of poverty	21.4	15.5	72.4	8.4
200% or more of poverty	148.3	132.3	89.2	71.4
Firm size of greatest earner				
Non-worker	27.0	20.7	76.7	11.2
Fewer than 10 employees	35.4	24.3	68.6	13.1
10-99 employees	43.4	33.5	77.2	18.1
100-499 employees	29.7	25.4	85.5	13.7
500 or more employees	90.6	81.3	89.7	43.9

Source: Employee Benefit Research Institute

Consumer price index for medical care

Exhibit 111. **Annual percentage change in selected components of the consumer price index**

	1981	1982	1983	1984	1985	1986	1987	1988	1989	1990	1991	1992	1993	1994
All items	10.3	6.2	3.2	4.3	3.6	1.9	3.6	4.1	4.8	5.4	4.2	3.0	3.0	2.6
All services	13.1	9.1	3.5	5.1	5.2	5.0	4.1	4.6	4.9	5.5	5.1	3.9	3.9	3.3
Medical care	10.7	11.7	8.7	6.3	6.2	7.6	6.6	6.5	7.6	9.1	8.6	7.4	5.4	4.8
Medical care commodities	11.0	10.3	8.6	7.3	7.2	6.5	6.7	6.9	7.8	8.4	8.2	6.4	3.7	2.9
Prescription drugs	11.4	11.6	11.0	9.6	9.5	8.6	8.1	7.9	8.7	10.0	9.9	7.5	3.9	3.4
Medical care services	10.7	12.0	8.7	6.0	6.1	7.7	6.6	6.4	7.7	9.3	8.9	7.6	6.5	5.2
Physician services	11.0	9.4	7.8	6.9	5.9	7.2	7.3	7.2	7.4	7.1	6.0	6.3	5.6	4.4
Hospital rooms	14.9	15.7	11.3	8.3	5.9	6.0	7.3	9.2	10.3	10.9	9.4	8.8	8.5	5.7

Source: US Bureau of Labor Statistics

Exhibit 112. **A comparison of inflation rates for all items and services, medical care services, physician servcies and hospital rooms**

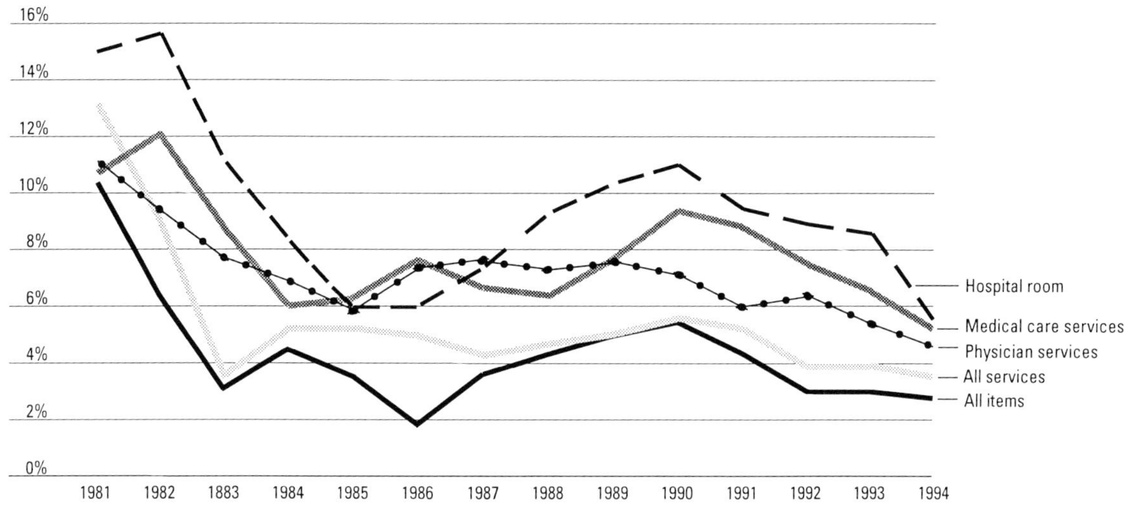

Source: US Bureau of Labor Statistics

List of sources

Exhibit

No.   Source

1   **Population**
Department of Commerce, Economics and Statistics Administration, Bureau of the Census, *Current Population Reports*, Series P25-1211, September 1994, and Series P25-1111, Tables 3 and 4, and Series P25-1018, Table 1, p. 1 and Table 6, p. 7 and Table G, p. 9, and Department of Health and Human Services, National Center for Health Statistics, Public Health Service, *Health, United States* (1993), Table 2, p. 61-62.

2   **International population**
Department of Commerce, Economics and Statistics Administration, Bureau of the Census, *Statistical Abstract of the United States* (1994), Comparative International Statistics—Introduction (p.839) and Table #1351 p.850-852.

3   **Life expectancy**
Department of Health and Human Services, National Center for Health Statistics, Public Health Service, *Monthly Vital Statistics Report* (Vol. 42, No. 13, October 11, 1994) Table 7, p. 17; Department of Health and Human Services, National Center for Health Statistics, Public Health Service, *Health, United States* (1993), Table 27, p. 91.

4   **International life expectancy**
Department of Health and Human Services, National Center for Health Statistics, Public Health Service, *Health, United States* (1993), Table 26, p.89-90.

5 **Birth rates**

Department of Health and Human Services, National Center for Health Statistics, Public Health Service, *Monthly Vital Statistics Report* (Vol. 43, No. 5, October 25, 1994) Table 1, p. 32; *Monthly Vital Statistics Report* (Vol. 42, No. 13, October 11, 1994) Table A, p. 2.

6 **Birth rates by age of mother**

Department of Health and Human Services, National Center for Health Statistics, Public Health Service, *Health, United States* (1993), Table 3, p.64; *Monthly Vital Statistics Report* (Vol. 43, No. 5, October 25, 1994) Table 3, p. 34.

7 **International birth rates**

Department of Commerce, Economics and Statistics Administration, Bureau of the Census, *Statistical Abstract of the United States* (1994), Table #1353 pp. 854-855.

8 **Infant mortality**

Department of Health and Human Services, National Center for Health Statistics, Public Health Service, *Monthly Vital Statistics Report* (Vol. 42, No. 13, October 11, 1994) Table 15, p. 31 and Table A, p. 2.

9 **International infant mortality**

Department of Health and Human Services, National Center for Health Statistics, Public Health Service, *Health, United States* (1993), Table 25, p. 88.

10 **Death rates**

Department of Health and Human Services, National Center for Health Statistics, Public Health Service, *Monthly Vital Statistics Report* (Vol. 42, No. 13, October 11, 1994) Table 5, p. 15.

11 **Leading causes of death**

Department of Health and Human Services, National Center for Health Statistics, Public Health Service, *Monthly Vital Statistics Report* (Vol. 42, No. 13, October 11, 1994) Table H, p. 7.

12   **Death rates by cause and race**

Department of Health and Human Services, National Center for Health Statistics, Public Health Service, *Health, United States* (1993), Tables 33-38, pp. 103-109.

13   **Notifiable disease rates**

Department of Health and Human Services, National Center for Health Statistics, Public Health Service, *Health, United States* (1993), Table 60, p. 142.

14   **Causes of death for infants**

Department of Health and Human Services, National Center for Health Statistics, Public Health Service, *Monthly Vital Statistics Report* (Vol. 43, No. 6, December 8, 1994) Table 26, p. 65.

15   **Vaccination rates for children**

Department of Health and Human Services, National Center for Health Statistics, Public Health Service, *Health, United States* (1993), Table 59, p. 141.

16   **Low birthweight**

Department of Health and Human Services, National Center for Health Statistics, Public Health Service, *Monthly Vital Statistics Report* (Vol. 43, No. 5(S), October 25, 1994) Table 43, p. 76.

17   **Teenage and unmarried mother births**

Department of Commerce, Economics and Statistics Administration, Bureau of the Census, *Statistical Abstract of the United States* (1994), Table 97, p. 79.

18   **International teenage mother births**

US Congress, Office of Technology Assessment, *International Health Statistics—What the Numbers Mean for the United States*, November 1993, Table 4.5, p. 41.

19   **Reported AIDS cases**

Department of Health and Human Services, National Center for Health Statistics, Public Health Service, *Health, United States* (1993), Table 61, p. 143; Centers for Disease Control National AIDS Clearinghouse, *AIDS Surveillance Report*, Year End Edition (1994), Table 1.

20   **Deaths from AIDS**

Department of Health and Human Services, National Center for Health Statistics, Public Health Service, *Health, United States* (1993), Table 61, p. 143; Centers for Disease Control National AIDS Clearinghouse, *AIDS Surveillance Report*, Year End Editions, 1991—Table 13, 1992—Table 13, 1994—Table 14.

21   **AIDS cases by state**

Centers for Disease Control National AIDS Clearinghouse, *AIDS Surveillance Report*, Year End Edition (1994), Table 1.

22   **AIDS cases and case fatality rates**

Centers for Disease Control National AIDS Clearinghouse, *AIDS Surveillance Report*, Year End Edition (1994), Table 13.

23   **Per capita ethanol consumption**

Department of Commerce, Economics and Statistics Administration, Bureau of the Census, *Statistical Abstract of the United States* (1994), Table 222, p. 148.

24   **Cigarette smoking among adults**

Department of Health and Human Services, National Center for Health Statistics, Public Health Service, *Health, United States* (1993), Table 72, p. 156.

25   **Drug use among high school seniors**

Johnston, Lloyd D., Patrick M. O'Malley, and Jerald G. Bachman, Department of Health and Human Services, *National Survey Results on Drug Use from the Monitoring the Future Study, 1975-1992* (1993).

26 **Crime victimization**
Bureau of Justice Statistics, Office of Justice Programs, Department of Justice, *Sourcebook of Criminal Justice Statistics* (1993), Table 3.1, p. 246 and Table 3.2, p. 247.

27 **Cost of AIDS, average annual cost**
Hellinger, Fred J., "The Lifetime Cost of Treating a Person with HIV," *Journal of the American Medical Association*, Vol. 270, No. 4, July 1993, Table 2, p. 476.

28 **Cost of AIDS by disease stage**
Hellinger, Fred J., "The Lifetime Cost of Treating a Person with HIV," *Journal of the American Medical Association*, Vol. 270, No. 4, July 1993, Table 3, p. 477.

29 **Cost of firearm injuries**
Max, Wendy and Dorothy Rice, "Shooting in the Dark: Estimating the Cost of Firearm Injuries," *Health Affairs*, Winter 1993, Exhibit 2, p. 177, and Exhibit 7, p. 181.

30 **Victim costs per injury**
Miller, Ted, Mark Cohen, and Shelli Rossman, "Victim Costs of Violent Crime and Resulting Injuries," *Health Affairs*, Winter 1993, Exhibit 3, p. 194.

31 **Lifetime costs of crime**
Miller, Ted, Mark Cohen, and Shelli Rossman, "Victim Costs of Violent Crime and Resulting Injuries," *Health Affairs*, Winter 1993, Exhibit 5, p. 195.

32 **Physicians per 100,000 population**
American Medical Association, *Physician Characteristics and Distribution in the US* (1994), Table A-16, p. 34.

33 **Physicians per 100,000 population by state**
American Medical Association, *Physician Characteristics and Distribution in the US* (1994), Table A-18, p. 38.

34 **Physician population by major activity and specialty**
American Medical Association, *Physician Characteristics and Distribution in the US* (1994), Table A-1, p. 19, Table A-17, p. 35, and Table A-2, p. 20.

35 **Physician population, demographics**
American Medical Association, *Physician Characteristics and Distribution in the US* 1994 edition— Table A-5, p. 23, Table A-6, p. 24, Table A-14, p. 32; 1993 edition—Table B-1, p. 47, Table A-9, p. 25, Table A-10, p. 26; 1987 edition—Table A-6, p.28.

36 **Physician population, projections**
Rivo, Marc L. and David Satcher, "Improving Access to Health Care," *Journal of the American Medical Association* (September 1993), Vol. 270, No. 9, Figure 4, p. 1077.

37 **Undergraduate medical school applications**
Jonas, Harry S., et al., " Educational Programs in US Medical Schools," *Journal of the American Medical Association* (September 1994), Vol. 272, No. 9, Table 4, p. 696.

38 **Undergraduate medical education**
Jonas, Harry S., et al., " Educational Programs in US Medical Schools," *Journal of the American Medical Association* (September 1994), Vol. 272, No. 9, Table 1, p. 695, Table 4, p. 696, and Table 9, p. 698.

39 **First-year medical students by race**
Jonas, Harry S., et al., " Educational Programs in US Medical Schools," *Journal of the American Medical Association* (September 1994), Vol. 272, No. 9, Table 8, p. 698.

40   **Graduate medical school enrollment**

Jonas, Harry S., et al., " Educational Programs in US Medical Schools," *Journal of the American Medical Association* (September 1994), Vol. 272, No. 9, Appendix II, Table 1, p. 698.

41   **Medical school expenses**

Krakower, Jack Y., et al., "US Medical School Finances," *Journal of the American Medical Association* (September 1993), Vol. 270, No. 9, Table 3, p. 1088.

42   **Loans and scholarship programs**

Krakower, Jack Y. et al., "US Medical School Finances," *Journal of the American Medical Association* (September 1993), Vol. 270, No. 9, Table 5 and 6, p. 1091; Ganem, Janice L. et al., "US Medical School Finances, 1992-1993," *Journal of the American Medical Association* (September 1994), Vol. 272, No. 9, Table 5, p. 711.

43   **Medical education indebtedness**

Kassebaum, David G. and Philip L. Szenas, "Relationship Between Indebtedness and the Specialty Choice of Graduating Medical Students," *Academic Medicine* (October 1992), Vol. 67, No. 10, Table 7, p. 705.

44   **Physician productivity measures**

American Medical Association, *Socioeconomic Characteristics of Medical Practice 1995*, Figure 1, p. 38 and Table 16, p. 72.

45   **Weeks practiced**

American Medical Association, *Socioeconomic Characteristics of Medical Practice*, 1995 edition—Table 2, p. 42; 1986 to 1995 editions—Table 1; Socioeconomic Monitoring System Database, 1985-1994.

46   **Practice hours per week**

American Medical Association, *Socioeconomic Characteristics of Medical Practice*, 1995 edition—Table 4, p. 46; 1986 to 1995 editions—Table 3; Socioeconomic Monitoring System Database, 1985-1994.

47   **Visits per week**

American Medical Association, *Socioeconomic Characteristics of Medical Practice*, 1995 edition—Table 16, p. 72; 1986 to 1995 editions—Table 15; Socioeconomic Monitoring System Database, 1985-1994.

48   **Days to schedule an appointment**

American Medical Association, Center for Health Policy Research, Socioeconomic Monitoring System, 1994.

49   **Waiting time**

American Medical Association, Center for Health Policy Research, Socioeconomic Monitoring System, 1983-1994.

50   **Physician-patient encounters**

American Medical Association, Center for Health Policy Research, *Policy Research Perspectives*, "An Estimate of Physician-Patient Encounters," (May 15, 1995), Table 1.

51   **Physician income and expenses**

American Medical Association, *Socioeconomic Characteristics of Medical Practice*, 1995 edition, Table 33, p. 112, Table 34, p. 114, and Table 48, p. 142; 1986 to 1995 editions—Tables 42 and 47; Socioeconomic Monitoring System, 1984-1994.

52   **Professional expenses**

American Medical Association, Center for Health Policy Research, *1994 Physician Survey*, Figure 4, p. 2.

53   **Expenses of self-employed physicians**

American Medical Association, *Socioeconomic Characteristics of Medical Practice*, 1995 edition—Table 33, p. 112, Table 34, p. 114; Socioeconomic Monitoring System, 1984-1994.

54   **Net income**

American Medical Association, *Socioeconomic Characteristics of Medical Practice*, 1995 edition—Table 48, p. 142; 1986 to 1995 editions—Tables 42 and 47; Socioeconomic Monitoring System, 1984-1994.

55   Liability claims per 100 physicians

American Medical Association, *Socioeconomic Characteristics of Medical Practice*, 1995 edition—Table 1, p. 32; Socioeconomic Monitoring System, 1985-1994.

56   Liability premiums

American Medical Association, *Socioeconomic Characteristics of Medical Practice*, 1995 edition—Table 1, p. 32; Socioeconomic Monitoring System, 1985-1994.

57   Change in professional liability expenses

American Medical Association, *Socioeconomic Characteristics of Medical Practice*, 1995 edition—Table 43, p. 130 and Table 44, p. 132; Socioeconomic Monitoring System, 1985-1994.

58   Frequent malpractice allegations

St. Paul Fire & Marine Insurance Company, *Physicians and Surgeons Update—Year End Report* (1994), 1994 Allegations Review section. **Reprinted with permission.

59   Costly malpractice allegations

St. Paul Fire & Marine Insurance Company, *Physicians and Surgeons Update—Year End Report* (1994), 1994 Allegations Review section. **Reprinted with permission.

60   Malpractice verdict awards

Jury Verdict Research, Inc., *Current Award Trends in Personal Injury, 1995 Edition*, *Medical Malpractice Chart*, p. 15. **Reprinted with permission.

61   Underwriting premiums and losses

A.M. Best Company, *Best's Aggregates and Averages, Property-Casualty 1993, Cumulative by Line Underwriting Experience-Industry*, p. 165, and *Industry Net Premiums Written by Lines of Business*, p. 180. **Reprinted with permission.

62 **Osteopathic physicians**

Department of Health and Human Services, Public Health Service, Health Resources and Services Administration, Bureau of Health Professions, *Seventh Report to the President and Congress on the Status of Health Personnel in the United States* (March 1990), Table VI-A-12, p. VI-45.

63 **Health care personnel**

Department of Health and Human Services, National Center for Health Statistics, Public Health Service, *Health, United States* (1993), Table 111, p. 204.

64 **Health professional school graduates**

Department of Health and Human Services, National Center for Health Statistics, Public Health Service, *Health, United States* (1993), Table 114, p. 208.

65 **Employment in medical-related industries**

Department of Labor, Bureau of Labor Statistics, *Employment and Earnings*, (August 1992 and September 1993), Table B-2, *Employees on Nonfarm Payrolls by Detailed Industry*.

66 **Hospital beds, admissions and outpatient visits**

American Hospital Association, *Hospital Statistics*, 1994-95 edition, Table 1, pp. 2-3. **Reprinted with permission.

67 **Growth in hospital utilization**

American Hospital Association, *Hospital Statistics*, 1994-95 edition, Table 1, pp. 2-3. **Reprinted with permission.

68 **Change in hospital utilization**

American Hospital Association, *Hospital Statistics*, 1994-95 edition, Table 1, pp. 2-3. **Reprinted with permission.

69 **Average length of stay**

American Hospital Association, *Hospital Statistics*, 1994-95 edition, Table 1, p. 3. **Reprinted with permission.

70 **Registered hospitals by characteristic**

American Hospital Association, *Hospital Statistics*, 1994-95 and 1982 editions—Tables 4A and 4B, p. 14-15, and 1972 edition—Table 4, p. 28 and Table 5, p. 34-52. **Reprinted with permission.

71 **For-profit hospitals and beds**

American Hospital Association, *Hospital Statistics*, 1994-95 edition, Table 1, p. 3. **Reprinted with permission.

72 **Growth in number of beds**

American Hospital Association, *Hospital Statistics*, 1994-95 edition, Table 1, p. 3. **Reprinted with permission.

73 **Growth in hospital beds by ownership and multihospital status**

American Hospital Association, *Guide to the Health Care Field*, 1993 edition, *Statistics for Multihospital Health Care Systems and Their Hospitals*, Table 3, p. B-3. **Reprinted with permission.

74 **Multihospital system members and beds**

American Hospital Association, *Guide to the Health Care Field*, 1983 to 1993 editions, *Statistics for Multihospital Health Care Systems and Their Hospitals*, Table 3, p. B-3.**Reprinted with permission.

75 **Unsponsored and uncompensated care**

US Congress, Congressional Budget Office, *A CBO Study: Trends in Health Spending—An Update* (June 1993), Table 2, p. 9.

76 **Real unsponsored and uncompensated care**

US Congress, Congressional Budget Office, *A CBO Study: Trends in Health Spending—An Update* (June 1993), Table A-10, p. 58.

77 **International comparisons of acute care hospitals and physicians**

American Medical Association, Center for Health Policy Research, *International Health Systems: A Chartbook Perspective* (1995), Chart 19, p. 24.

78 **International comparisons of acute hospital beds and employees**
American Medical Association, Center for Health Policy Research, *International Health Systems: A Chartbook Perspective* (1995), Chart 30, p. 36.

79 **Physicians with managed care contracts**
American Medical Association, *Socioeconomic Characteristics of Medical Practice*, 1995 edition- Table 2, p. 5.

80 **Revenue from managed care contracts**
American Medical Association, *Socioeconomic Characteristics of Medical Practice*, 1995 edition- Table 4, p. 7.

81 **Capitation and withholds**
American Medical Association, *Socioeconomic Characteristics of Medical Practice*, 1995 edition- Table 6, p. 8.

82 **Operational PPOs by ownership**
Marion Merrell Dow, *Managed Care Digest—PPO Edition, 1994, Industry Summary Chart*, p. 4. and SMG Marketing Group. **Reprinted with permission.

83 **Growth of HMOs**
Managed Care Outlook (December 16, 1994) Vol. 7, No. 24, *HMO Enrollment Tops 50 Million*, p. 5.; InterStudy, *The InterStudy Edge, Managed Care: A Decade in Review 1980-1990*, pp. 65-66; and *Statistical Abstract of the United States*, 1987 edition, Table 138, p. 90. **Reprinted with permission.

84 **State penetration of HMOs**
Managed Care Outlook (June 17, 1994) Vol. 7, No. 12, *Number of HMOs and Enrollees by State Year-End 1993*, p. 5. **Reprinted with permission.

85   Managed care market share

American Medical Association, Center for Health Policy Research, *Physician Marketplace Trends Presentation* (October 1994, *Managed Care Market Share: 1988 and 1993*, p. 2.

86   Employee enrollment in health plans

Foster Higgins, *National Survey of Employer-Sponsored Health Plans* (February 1995), as abridged in *Medical Benefits* (March 15, 1995). Vol. 12, No. 5, *Figure 1. Distribution of Employee Enrollment in Employer-Sponsored Health Plans by Plan Type, 1992 to 1994*, p. 1. **Reprinted with permission.

87   Monthly premium costs

Managed Care Outlook (March 10, 1995) Vol. 8, No. 5, *1995 Average Monthly Cost Levels by Type of Plan*, p. 1. **Reprinted with permission.

88   Growth in health insurance premiums

KPMG Peat Marwick LLP, *Health Benefits in 1994* (October 1994), as abridged in *Medical Benefits* (November 15, 1994), Vol. 11, No. 21, *Figure 1. Rate of Increase in Health Premiums, 1991 to 1994*, p. 1. **Reprinted with permission.

89   National health expenditures as a percent of GDP

Levit, Katharine, et al., Department of Health and Human Services, Health Care Financing Administration, "National Health Expenditures, 1993," *Health Care Financing Review* (Fall 1994), Vol. 16, No. 1, Table 11, p. 280; and US Congress, Congressional Budget Office, *CBO Memorandum—Projections of National Health Expenditures,1993 Update*, Table 1, p. 2.

90   Nation's health dollar

Levit, Katharine, et al., Department of Health and Human Services, Health Care Financing Administration, "National Health Expenditures, 1993," *Health Care Financing Review* (Fall 1994), Vol. 16, No. 1, Figure 2, p. 252.

91   **Personal health care expenditures by source**
Levit, Katharine, et al., Department of Health and Human Services, Health Care Financing Administration, "National Health Expenditures, 1993," *Health Care Financing Review* (Fall 1994), Vol. 16, No. 1, Table 13, pp. 283-284.

92   **National health expenditures: Amount, growth and percent of GDP**
Levit, Katharine, et al., Department of Health and Human Services, Health Care Financing Administration, "National Health Expenditures, 1993," *Health Care Financing Review* (Fall 1994), Vol. 16, No. 1, Table 11, p. 280.

93   **Regional differences in health care expenditures**
Vincenzino, Joseph V., *Statistical Bulletin* (January-March 1995), as abridged in *Medical Benefits* (February 15, 1995), Vol. 12, No. 3, *Table 2. Per Capita Health Care Expenditures, by Region, 1991,* p. 4. **Reprinted with permission.

94   **National health expenditures by type of expenditure**
Levit, Katharine, et al., Department of Health and Human Services, Health Care Financing Administration, "National Health Expenditures, 1993," *Health Care Financing Review* (Fall 1994), Vol. 16, No. 1, Table 12, p. 281.

95   **Projections of national health expenditures**
US Congress, Congressional Budget Office, *CBO Memorandum—Projections of National Health Expenditures,1993 Update*, Table 1, p. 2, and Table 2, p. 3.

96   **International health expenditures comparisons**
Murray, CJL, R. Govindaraj, and P. Musgraove, "National Health Expenditures: A Global Analysis," *Bulletin of the World Health Organization*, Vol. 72, No. 4, *Annex Table: Total Health Expenditures: Public, Private and Aid Flows*, p. 635.

97   **Health insurance primary coverage enrollment**
US Congress, Congressional Budget Office, *CBO Memorandum—Projections of National Health Expenditures, 1993 Update*, Table A-9, p. 17.

98   Medicare and Medicaid public expenditures

Department of Health and Human Services, Health Care Financing Administration, *HHS News, National Health Expenditures Press Release* (November 11, 1994), Table 3—*Personal Health Care Expenditures by Type of Expenditure and Selected Sources of Payment: Calendar Year 1993* and 1992 HCFA figures were provided by personnel communication.

99   Medicaid recipients and payments

Department of Health and Human Services, Social Security Administration, *Social Security Bulletin, Annual Statistical Supplement, 1993*, Table 8.E2, p. 320.

100   Medicare per capita reimbursement

Department of Health and Human Services, Health Care Financing Administration, Bureau of Data Management and Strategy, Office of Statistics and Data Management, *1993 Preliminary Annual Summary Controls.*

101   Medicare enrollees and outlays

US Congress, Congressional Budget Office, Committee on Ways and Means., *Green Book, 1994,* Table 5-20, p. 176. and US Department of Health and Human Services, Health Care Financing Administration, *Health Care Financing Review: Medicare and Medicaid Statistical Supplement*, Table 5, p.155.

102   Medicaid payments—total and per eligible recipient

Department of Health and Human Services, Social Security Administration, *Social Security Bulletin: Annual Statistical Supplement, 1993*, Table 8.E1, p. 319.

103   Medicare benefit payments

Department of Health and Human Services, Social Security Administration, *Social Security Bulletin: Annual Statistical Supplement, 1993*, Table 8.A1, p. 302, and Table 8.A2, p. 303.

104 **Distribution of Medicare reimbursements**
Department of Health and Human Services, Social Security Administration, *Social Security Bulletin: Annual Statistical Supplement, 1993*, Table 8.B1, p. 304, and Table 8.B2, p. 305.

105 **Medicare enrollee costs—table**
US Congress, Congressional Budget Office, Committee on Ways and Means., *Green Book, 1994,* Table B-7, pp. 876-877.

106 **Medicare enrollee costs—chart**
US Congress, Congressional Budget Office, Committee on Ways and Means., *Green Book, 1994,* Table B-7, pp. 876-877.

107 **Medicare enrollment and payments according to survival status**
Lubitz, James D. and Gerald F. Riley, "Trends in Medicare Payments in the Last Year of Life," *The New England Journal of Medicine*, Vol. 328, No. 15 (April 15, 1993), Table 1, p. 1093. **Reprinted with permission.

108 **Medicare payments in last year of life**
Lubitz, James D. and Gerald F. Riley., "Trends in Medicare Payments in the Last Year of Life," *The New England Journal of Medicine*, Vol. 328, No. 15 (April 15, 1993), Figure 1, p. 1095. **Reprinted with permission.

109 **Characteristics of the uninsured**
Employee Benefit Research Institute, *Sources of Health Insurance and Characteristics of the Uninsured: Analysis of the March 1994 Current Population Survey*, EBRI Special Report SR-28, Issue Brief No. 158, February 1995, Tables 14 and 15. **Reprinted with permission.

110 **Characteristics of the insured**
Employee Benefit Research Institute, *Sources of Health Insurance and Characteristics of the Uninsured: Analysis of the March 1994 Current Population Survey*, EBRI Special Report SR-28, Issue Brief No. 158, February 1995, Tables 14 and 15. **Reprinted with permission.

111 **Annual percentage changes in the CPI**

American Medical Association, Center for Health Policy Research, "Consumer Price Index: 1994 Year-End Report," Table 1, p.2.

112 **Comparison of inflation rates**

American Medical Association, Center for Health Policy Research, "Consumer Price Index: 1994 Year-End Report," Table 1, p.2.

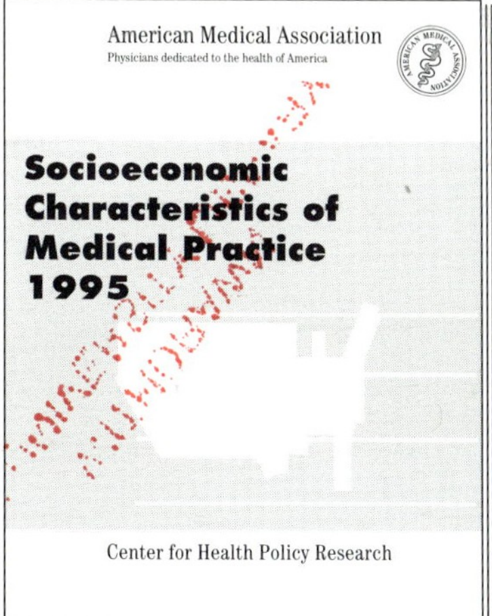

Get a comprehensive view of US medical practice

For sophisticated statistical research and analysis of the socioeconomic aspects of current medical practice, rely on the publications of the AMA Center for Health Policy Research. Data is derived from the annual AMA Socioeconomic Monitoring System survey program.

Providing a valuable overview...

Socioeconomic Characteristics of Medical Practice, 1995
Comprehensive, timely and easy-to-use, this important reference book provides a definitive profile of US medical practice. It includes data on many measures of medical practice, such as physician earnings, work patterns and fees. Annual, published April.
Order #: OP192695 Price: $114.95.

Phone orders 800 621-8335

American Express, Visa, MasterCard and Optima accepted. Handling charges and local taxes apply.